I0559678

# Sex in Sobriety

A Qualitative Narrative Exploration of the Utilization
of Mindfulness Practices for Enjoyable Sober Sex

2nd Edition 2025

# Dr. Anadel Baughn Barbour

*This is dedicated to all the sober people that have gone before me who suffered so much fear that they never found a way to enjoy sex in sobriety. This is dedicated to those who have joined me in sobriety to find ways to have better sex lives in sobriety. Finally this is dedicated to all the sober people that come after me, that they find peace through Mindfulness and enjoyable sex in sobriety.*

# Foreword

It has been eight years since the first printing of this book in April 2017. I am very happy for any help it has provided. I am pleased to report that the subjects of the research reported positive changes in their lives. I would also like to clarify that, although the effects of substances and mindfulness practices on the body and mind have not changed, the types of substances, as well as their accessibility, potency, and availability, have evolved. This foreword will bring currency to the new release of this text.

I am happy to report that I have been in contact with all the subjects in my study, and as of last year, the results were positive. Each subject reported continued sobriety and lasting benefits of mindfulness practices in their relationships over the past seven years. Subjects #1 and #3 reported higher self-esteem, with #3 expressing more courage in approaching sex partners. Subject #2 reported fewer arguments with their partner and a reduction in anxiety before and during sex. Subject #4 reported increased self-confidence, noting that the ability to initiate sex was the most enjoyable benefit of mindfulness.

New and more potent drugs have emerged since the first printing of this text. In the *Depressant Category*, *Fentanyl* stands out as the most detrimental substance to emerge in quite some time and has become rampant in our society. Bought on the street or the Dark Web, it is highly addictive and more deadly than its opioid counterparts. In the *Stimulant Category, ADHD Medications such as Ritalin, Adderall, and*

*Vyvanse* are on the rise. There are more diagnoses of ADD/ADHD, both from doctors and from individuals who self-diagnose using WebMD. These stimulants are now more popular among students, who often access the drugs from peers with prescriptions. Overuse and abuse are, therefore, on the rise.

Devices have become a pervasive part of our society, bringing with them a new form of addiction. Internet addiction, including pornography and social media addiction, affects the brain much like stimulants do, and can cause significant damage to mental, physical, emotional, and spiritual health. Since abstinence from the World Wide Web and smartphones is not a realistic option, individuals must learn to use devices more productively and positively.

One positive result of widespread internet and device use is the easier access to *Mindfulness Practices*. Meditation and Mindfulness Applications such as *Calm, Mindfulness*, and *Insight Timer* make it simple to practice anywhere, at any time. Easier access to meditation teachers—from *Tara Brach to Pema Chödrön*—as well as to yoga teachings, from *Yin Yoga to Kundalini Yoga to Tantric practices*, can be found on YouTube and various websites and can be practiced in the privacy of one's own home.

I hope this book continues to help individuals on their journey to recovery, to find enjoyment in their sex lives, and to serve as an academic text for professors, teachers, and counselors in rehabilitation centers, as well as an educational tool for newly sober individuals seeking another way to live and enjoy their lives.

**My wish for you all:**

*May you be free from fear.*

*May you have mental happiness.*

*May you have physical happiness.*

*May you live with ease.*


With ease,

Anadel

# Acknowledgments

I would like to acknowledge my husband Christopher, for without whom I would never have experienced enjoyable sober sex. I would like to acknowledge Dr. Patti Britton, whose brilliant mind and loving spirit carried me through this amazing journey. I would like to acknowledge Dr. Robert Dunlap whose knowledge and tenderness led me in the right direction. And finally, I want to acknowledge Dr. Stephanie Hunter Jones, for without her bright spirit shining alongside of me, and her unwavering support, I would never have found this road to take.

# About the Author

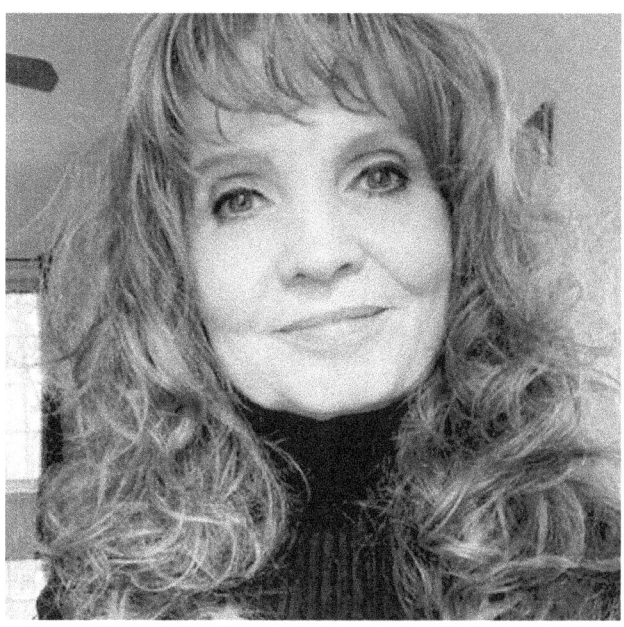

My story, with its unwritten chapters of poverty and neglect, mental illness and addictions, led me to exactly where I am supposed to be. Every difficulty and misfortune made me who I am and led me to do what I do right here, right now. At the age of 40, with a High School education, a slew of failed relationships and unattained career goals, I bottomed out, felt a glimmer of hope and got help! Because my life has been filled with challenges, I have a deep understanding of suffering. My journey to here was made up of years of family dysfunction and abuse, drug and alcohol addiction, mad passion for acting and punk rock, and many failed loves and lusts. My life changed when I decided to do things differently. I got sober. I began to heal.

As my body and mind began to heal, new goals began to develop. With much support from Spiritual teachers, therapists and mentors, I jumped onto the road of recovery and self-discovery: 12 Steps, Mindful practices, school, spiritual quests, higher education, and finally, I found my purpose and now my passion: Helping people heal their minds, bodies, spirits. I love being a Mindful EMDR Therapist. Seeing people transform their fear into calmness is the greatest reward I get from the work I do.

And I still love punk rock and acting!

# Abstract

This Qualitative Narrative study explores the lived experiences of four sober individuals who had negative experiences during sober sex and later applied Mindfulness practices that improved the quality of their sober sexual experiences. Pertinent literature about the mind-altering substances of marijuana, stimulants, depressants and alcohol are reviewed with historical references to their origins, information about physical, emotional, mental and spiritual effects to the brain and nervous system, focusing on the body, mind and effects on sex. The origins of Mindfulness are reviewed, followed by details of the physical, psychological and spiritual effects that Mindful meditation and yoga practices have on the brain and the nervous system, focusing on the body, mind and effects on sex. Results were obtained from narratives and answers to questionnaires provided by the participants using the Labovian Structure Method. Dissemination of the narratives determined the efficacy of applying Mindfulness to sober sex as a solution to improving sex in recovery. Findings showed sober sex was more enjoyable for sober individuals who practiced Mindful mediation and yoga. Further exploration is needed to open dialogue with professionals in the recovery and sexology fields to add Mindfulness to their discussions and treatments for sober sexual concerns.

# Chapter 1 - Introduction

## The Focus: Sex in Sobriety

The path to sober sex is complex. For those with a history of substance abuse who have achieved sobriety and follow Mindfulness and yoga practices, the results may be worth the journey for a sex life that is enjoyable. This study is about that journey. Using a sample of those who have incorporated Mindfulness meditation and yoga practices in their recovery, the focus is on the substances that impact sexual function and pleasure, and the possibility that Mindfulness meditation and yoga practices can improve recovery for a better sexual experience overall.

Despite the large volume of empirical research about treatment for addiction, the subject of sober sex is limited. There are volumes of empirical research about Mindfulness practices including evidence that meditation and yoga affect actual changes to the brain. The need for continued exploration in the complexity of sober sex and the use of Mindfulness practices, as a means for enjoyable sober sex is the inspiration for this study.

This Qualitative Narrative research study will explore the lived experience of four sober individuals that will include reflections, observations and descriptions of sexual experiences during life before recovery, once sobriety was achieved and finally after the utilization of Mindfulness practices during sober sex.

The study will be important for professionals in the field of recovery to begin to understand the challenges that arise for sober individuals in relation to sex. It will create an open dialogue about an area of recovery that has been ignored in treatment facilities.

The study provides a viable solution to overcoming emotional blocks and physical limitations that have kept many sober people from enjoying sex.

## The Problem

Sex in sobriety can be quite frightening. In an interview by Rapkin (2014), actor Colin Farrell revealed:

I made love to a woman about two and a half years after I got clean and sober and it was one of the most terrifying moments of my life. It was in the afternoon. The windows and the curtains were open. It was lovely and to be crass it wasn't fucking. She was very gentle. But it was terrifying. Because I was just used to drunkenness and dark rooms and clubs and toilets and whatever. (www.elle.com, n/p)

The problem was shown to be the need for a solution to overcome the fear of sober sex.

Research has shown the ability to enjoy sex comes from being aware and present. The road to present-time awareness comes with the Mindfulness practices of meditation and yoga. The discovery of how to engage in enjoyable sober sex through Mindfulness practices gave rise to this study.

The study explored of the sex lives of sober alcoholics and addicts who also practiced Mindfulness. The focus of the study was to find out if sex in sobriety had become more enjoyable for them after the utilization and application of Mindfulness techniques. Kettlehack (1993) captured the essence of the problem:

Sobriety is an astonishing revelatory, wonderful gift; few recovering alcoholics and drug addicts who've managed to stay sober for any length of time would disagree with this. But despite our newfound clarity, few of us escape having problems with sex, intimacy and love...we experience some of our greatest blocks in the sexual arena because, for most of us, sex requires a degree of nakedness (psychic as well as physical) that few recovering people are willing to experience without the buffering, muting, fantasizing effects of drugs and alcohol. (p. 3)

Kettlehack (1993) concluded that for those who use and abuse drugs, sexual encounters presented challenges. Unable to face social setting without being altered, addicts and alcoholics believed that they needed to be high or drunk to enjoy sex (Braun-Harvey, 2009, p. 2). Many of those experiences have left the individual filled with guilt and shame. Alcoholics Anonymous (1952) described the emotional life of a newly sober alcoholic in this way: Very deep, sometimes quite forgotten, damaging emotional conflicts persist below the level of consciousness. At the time of these occurrences, they may actually have given our emotions violent twists which have since discolored our personalities and altered our lives for the worse. (p. 79-80)

Although sobriety began with abstinence from a mind-altering substance, recovery required more than abstinence from drugs and alcohol. There persisted emotional damage deep within the mind of a person in recovery. Anger and mistrust were present in many a newly sober individual, causing difficulty in relationships with others. As Alcoholics Anonymous (1952) explained:

Resentment is the "number" one offender. It destroys more alcoholics than anything else. From it stem all forms of spiritual disease for we have been not only mentally and physically ill, we have been spiritually sick. When the spiritual malady is overcome, we straighten out mentally and physically. (p. 64)

Much of the ability to remain sober comes from soul searching and building a strong spiritual foundation. Alcoholics Anonymous (1952) continued, "The spiritual life is not a theory. We *have to live it*" (p. 83).Reparation during recovery is in large part internal. Mindful meditation practices provide a doorway into the mind. Mindful yoga practices provide a bridge to physical health. Practicing meditation and yoga embodies mind and spirit. This study revealed that combining them with sober sex was found to ease the fears and bring pleasure to sober sexual experiences.

The minimum amount of empirical evidence on this subject created an opportunity to research a connection between Mindfulness practices and sex in sobriety. First, literature was reviewed that detailed the effects of mind-altering substances on the body, the mind and the spirit. Scientific perspectives and psychological perspectives provided historical data about mind-altering substances and the effects that led to difficult sexual practices (Braun-Harvey, 2009, p. 7). The researcher then reviewed literature explaining scientific and psychological perspectives about the effects of meditation and yoga on the body, mind and spirit. Next, a study was conducted with a small sample providing narratives detailing their lived-experiences of combining Mindfulness practices with sex in sobriety.

## Purpose of the Study

The purpose of the study was to show how Mindfulness practices could benefit people in recovery to find pleasure and enjoyment in their sex lives. By gathering information through the lived experiences of people in recovery, the sample provided details about sex before sobriety, sex in early sobriety before practicing Mindfulness, and finally their experiences after combining Mindfulness practices to sexual practices.

Living a sober lifestyle requires deliberate changes to behavior (Levine, 2007, p. 101). That includes deliberate changes to thoughts and intentions. Mindful meditation stills the mind. Mindful yoga elevates energy, and contributes to better physical health. Combining meditation and yoga creates a connection between the mind and the body providing present-time awareness. Present-time awareness is an important component to enjoyable sober sex. Having found little empirical evidence to support the theory that a sober person could combine Mindful practices with sexual practices, exploration of the lived experiences of adult sober individuals was done. By having compared lived experiences of people in recovery who also practice

Mindful meditation and yoga, a conclusion was drawn about the effectiveness of combining sober sex and Mindfulness.

## Research Questions

Living a sober life means finding new ways to have fun, to create meaningful relationships and to experience enjoyable sex with another person. A number of questions arose during the research.

1) How do sober adults recall their sexual experiences while they were still using mind-altering substances?

2) How did getting sober change their sexual experiences?

3) What details can sober adults provide regarding changes in their sex lives after applying Mindfulness practices?

## Methodology

The method chosen for the study was a Qualitative approach using a narrative design with open-ended questions and interviews. According to Creswell (2014), "Narrative research is a design of inquiry from the humanities in which the researcher studies the lives of individuals and asks one or more individuals to provide stories about their lives" (p.13). This study has examined the lives of four sober people who have practiced Mindful meditation and yoga and have used it as a tool for better sex. The subjects were given a questionnaire that asked for their age, length of sobriety, and length of time they had been practicing Mindfulness. The subjects then reflected, in a narrative, their personal stories about sex before they were sober, after they got sober, and what changes occurred after introducing Mindful meditation and yoga practices into their sex lives. The setting for the study was each subject's home. Interviews were done in person and over the telephone, with written questionnaires and responses sent via e-fax and e-mail. To complete the study, final analyses entailed combining the experiences of the sample in a collaborative narrative.

## Rationale and Significance

The study was necessary on the professional level because very little research exists regarding sober sex. Studies for the treatment of addicts and alcoholics have covered abstinence from drugs and alcohol, using psycho-education for improving social skills, communication skills and nutritional guidance, ignoring education on sex, sexuality and sexual health. As described by Braun-Harvey (2009):

The current neglect of sexuality as a core issue in addiction recovery reflects the experience I had in 1982. I still have a vivid memory of the presentation about "Sex and Violence: The Unmentionable in Addiction Treatment." The responses from the attendees ranged from discomfort to anger. Many told me that their clients would relapse if these topics were discussed and that their clients were "not ready" for this work. I tried to explain that clients were at risk of relapse if we *did not* discuss these issues. (p. iv)

Although HIV and sexually transmitted diseases were discussed in treatment centers, he consistently found sober sex education to be excluded. Braun-Harvey, (2009) continued:

Recovery means more than the elimination of one's drug of choice, either through harm reduction or abstinence. Recovery is also about what is added or gained in one's life. To me, recovery means wholeness. It means having one's inner self, (thoughts, feelings, values, and beliefs) *connected and congruent* with one's outer self (behavior and relationships). Developing sexual health in recovery is essential to becoming an integrated, whole person. (p. 32)

This study was necessary to individuals in recovery who have longed to enjoy sex while living a sober life.

## Role of the Researcher

The role of the researcher was that of being a participant in the study, which could bring inherent concerns to the study. As Creswell (2014) explained, "With these concerns in mind, inquirers explicitly identify reflexively their biases, values, and personal background" (p. 187). The commonality of sober sex combined with Mindful meditation and yoga would be the basis for the researcher's role in the study. As such, bias of outcome needed to be monitored. Values may have differed between subjects and researcher. A non-judging and non-shaming stance was necessary while conducting the interviews with participants.

As the researcher was not present for any of the subjects' actual sexual encounters, reliability of narratives depended on truthful answers from the participants in the sample.

## Researcher's Assumptions

The researcher has experience in bringing Mindfulness practices and sexual practices together with much success. The assumption that other sober individuals would have the same or similar experiences became the reason for the study.

Since the narratives of the subjects may or may not have reflected those of the researcher, questionnaires and subsequent interviews were conducted using open-ended questions as not to influence the subjects' responses.

## Definition of Terms

### Terms in Mind-Altering Substances Section

• Anhedonia: Inability to feel pleasure

• BAC's: Blood Alcohol Levels.

• Benzodiazepines: Refers to a class of drugs that have a sedative effect, and thus, are often used to successfully alleviate anxiety. These drugs are often referred to as tranquilizers. Popular benzodiazepines include Valium, Xanax, and Ativan.

• Biphasic: Having two phases

•Mind-Altering Substance: Consciousness-altering drug, psychoactive drug

• Neurotransmitter: Chemical substance that is released at the end of a nerve fiber by the arrival of a nerve impulse and, by diffusing across the synapse or junction, causes the transfer of the impulse to another nerve fiber, a muscle fiber, or some other structure.

• Sober Sex: Engaging in sexual activities without being altered by alcohol or drugs

• Wernicke-Korsakoff Syndrome: A brain disorder due to thiamine (vitamin B1) deficiency. Lack of vitamin B1 is common in people with alcoholism.

## Terms in the Mindfulness Practices Section

• Amygdala: a roughly almond-shaped mass of gray matter inside each cerebral hemisphere, involved with the experiencing of emotions.

• Asana: Sanskrit word for Pose

• EEG, also known as Electroencephalograph: a test or record of brain activity produced by electroencephalography.

• Lotus Position: A seated, cross-legged position used in yoga, meditation,

• MRI, also known as Magnetic Resonance Imaging: a pain-free non-invasive medical test used to produce two-dimensional images of the structures of the body. The process uses intense magnetic fields to make images of the inside of the body.

• Mindfulness: The act of paying attention in the moment without judgment.

• Neuroimaging: Scientific term used when images of the brain are obtained through MRI or EEG.

• Pranayama: Sanskrit word for Breath Control.

• Resourcing: Ways to cultivate self-regulation and evoke positive states of well-being.

• Yama: Sanskrit word for Restraint

• Yin Yoga: Practicing asanas that are held for long periods of time (3 minutes or more)

• Yoga: Sanskrit word for yoke. Uniting the breath with the body. Yoga practice combines movement of the body into an asana and control of the breath during the movement.

## In Conclusion

In the following chapters, information about marijuana, stimulants, depressants and alcohol were outlined from their origins to their effects on the human body, mental health and sex life. Detailed information about the beginnings of Mindfulness and the expansive nature of meditation and yoga in the spiritual realm as well as the scientific and psychological field followed, ending with the benefits of these practices to the body, mind, spirit and sexual satisfactions. Answers to questionnaires and brief narratives from the subjects were recorded in the fourth chapter, with collaborative narratives and findings included. Finally, pros and cons were debated, culminating in the results and possibilities for expanded future research on the topic of combining sober sex and Mindfulness.

# Chapter 2 - Literature Review

## Introduction

In order to answer the question of how Mindfulness practices could help sober individuals engage in enjoyable sex, inquiries for the lived experiences of individuals rather than measured or psychoanalytical methods of research were conducted. A qualitative narrative research method has been chosen, with information to be provided by four sober individuals who also practice Mindfulness.

It was important to understand how the brain worked since both drugs and Mindfulness practices affected the brain. In brief, as described by Kirsch (2010):

> The human brain contains about 100 billion nerve cells called neurons...Neurons do not actually touch each other. Rather there are fluid-filled gaps, called 'synapses' between the end of one and the beginning of another...chemicals called 'neurotransmitters,' which are manufactured by neurons, convey information across the gaps (that is synapses). Serotonin is one of the neurotransmitters...others include norepinephrine and dopamine. (p. 82)

The brain is an organ and it grows and matures along with the body. As Siegel (1999) reported, "At birth, the brain is the most undifferentiated organ in the body. Genes and early experience shape the way neurons connect to one another and thus form the specialized circuits that give rise to mental processes" (p. 14).

According to Siegel (2013), there occurred a growth spurt in the brain from age 12 to 24 (p. 6), and that "Brain changes during early teen years set up four qualities of our minds during adolescence: novelty seeking, social engagement, increased emotional intensity and creative exploration" (p. 7). He was describing that period of growth where thoughts, emotions, decision-making and personal interactions began to take shape. Those experiences, whether positive or negative, created pathways in the brain, which created values and ideals in the mind. Since experimentation with mind-altering substances usually began in early adolescence (Siegel, 2013, p. 75), brain development could be affected and could alter the natural changes in an adolescent brain. (p. 7).

It has been theorized that sexuality begins in childhood. Consider the findings as reported by Constantine and Martinson (1981) that, "Adult sexuality is intimately linked with child sexuality, not a sudden emergent consequence of physical development at puberty" (p. x). As reported by Steinhardt (2004), "A passionate advocate of education as prevention, [Mary] Calderone held that children should learn basic facts about sexuality as early as kindergarten" (c250.columbia.edu, n/p). Since sexuality was part of human nature, positive sex education and nurturing was vital to the development of healthy sexual values.

A reasonable conclusion could be made that using mind-altering substances during childhood and adolescence could affect chemical changes to the brain, creating emotional distortions in the mind resulting in unhealthy sexual experiences lasting into adulthood.

The first section reviewed literature that provides information on mind-altering substances, and their effects on individuals. The mind-altering substances studied were marijuana, stimulants, depressants, and alcohol. The research focused on each substance with information about its history and current trends in its use. The physical, emotional, mental, and spiritual effects were reviewed, including the serious affects from abuse that have created negative consequences to human sexuality and healthy sex lives for both men and women.

The second section reviewed literature about the Mindfulness practices of meditation and yoga. The review began with a brief history of each and continued with changes in the brain, mind states, breath, body and emotions that have been recorded by those who practice Mindfulness meditation and yoga along with the effects of applying the practices to affect changes to the sex lives of people in recovery (Braun-Harvey, 2009, p. 8).

## Mind-Altering Substances

The information contained in this research was derived from books, articles, scientific journals, and Government websites. Information was gathered from various authors, including Dr. Daniel J. Siegel, whose studies about the links between Mindfulness and the brain have brought legitimacy to the physical and emotional benefits of meditation, and Dr. Jon Kabat-Zinn, who pioneered the movement of bringing Mindfulness to the masses to relieve stress and pain, and from sites such as The National Institute on Drug Abuse, and The Institute for The Advancement of Human Sexuality. The research provided information on effects that mind-altering substances have on the brain, the body and the psyche, including sex and intimacy.

The term mind altering is defined as "causing marked changes in patterns of mood and behavior, as an hallucinogenic drug" (dictionary.reference.com, n/p). According to The Free Dictionary, (n/d), mind-altering substances were "consciousness-altering drug, psychoactive drug, psychoactive substance" (www.thefreedictionary.com, n/p).

Taking mind-altering substances was not necessarily a problem. Opiates have been used to relieve unbearable pain for cancer patients (Joranson, 1990, p.12-24). Marijuana has been found to reduce tension (Earleywine, 2002, p. 18). Alcohol has consistently been linked to religious ceremonies. (Phillips, 2014, p. 45). Stimulants were found to reduce activity in hyperactive children (Rasmussen, 2008, p. 231). Problems arose when intake of drugs and alcohol exceeded its usefulness and its enjoyment level (Kuhn, Swartzwelder and Wilson, 2008, p. 274). Substance abuse resulted in negative consequences including addiction. From failed relationships, to automobile accidents and even permanent psychosis, the negative consequences affected every area of the abuser's life (Nation Institute on Drug Abuse (NIDA), www.drugabuse.gov, n/p).

**Marijuana**

A natural plant substance, Marijuana has been found to have calming and hallucinatory qualities, which has made it an attractive substance for centuries. According to Kuhn, et al., (2008), "The first written accounts of cannabis cultivation appear in Chinese records

15

from as far back as 28 B. C., though the plant was likely cultivated for thousands of years before that" (p. 144). Considered either a gateway to harder drugs or harmless and natural, its popularity continues to rise. Medicinal uses included treatments for Glaucoma, cessation of nausea associated with Cancer treatments, appetite stimulation for wasting symptoms associated with HIV and AIDS, and more recently as treatment for anxiety and chronic pain relief (NIDA, www.drugabuse.gov, 2015, n/p).

Although still considered an illegal substance to consume and sell on the Federal level, many states have adopted laws that allow marijuana to be sold for medicinal purposes from local licensed shops. As Room (2014) explained:

In November 2012, voters in Colorado and Washington State voted for the state to set up a legal market in cannabis for non-medical use. It is expected that other US states, with provisions made for populace, will vote on similar measures in November 2014 and at the presidential election in November 2016. (p. 345-346)

**Physical Effects**

Including Tetrahydrocannabinols (THC), "Marijuana contains more than 460 active chemicals and over 60 unique cannabinoids" (Seamon, Fass, Maniscalco-Feichtl, & Abu-Shraie, 2007, p. 1038). The various methods of intake into the body were as follows: smoking a rolled cigarette (a joint), inhaling through a water pipe (a bong), inhaling with a vaporizer, eating it, dabbing the extracted resin (inhaling a dab of heated resin from a solid surface such as aluminum foil or a nail head) and as an edible (in baked goods such as cookies or brownies) (NIDA, www.drugabuse.gov, 2015, n/p). The initial feeling has been described as euphoria. Human physiology contributed to the fascination with marijuana's effects. Research has shown that the human brain has cannabanoid receptors (CB's) and as Seamon, et al., (2007), reported:

The effects of inhaled marijuana can be felt immediately. THC, a cannabinoid, passes rapidly from the lungs into the bloodstream to a number of body organs...CB1 receptors are present mainly in the central nervous system (CNS) and to a lesser extent in the peripheral tissue. CB1 receptors have a heterogeneous distribution pattern in the brain, which account for the myriad of marijuana's effects on pleasure, memory, thought, concentration, sensory and time perception, and coordinated movement. (p. 1038)

As reported by Kuhn, et al. (2008), the hippocampus, being most directly affected by marijuana intake, is the area of the brain involved in the formation of memories which explains why marijuana abusers appear forgetful. Kuhn, et al., (2008) revealed, "[The hippocampus] has a very high concentration of cannabanoid receptors. Not surprisingly, the inhibition of memory formation by marijuana is its most well-established negative effect on mental function" (p. 150). They found that smoking marijuana did not immediately affect breathing, although it directly affected the lungs, causing a decrease in their capacity to hold air (Kuhn, et al., 2008, p. 152).

NIDA (2015) reported, "Contrary to common belief, marijuana can be addictive. Research suggests that about 1 in 11 users become addicted to marijuana. This number increases among those who start as teens (to about 17 percent, or 1 in 6) and among people who use marijuana daily (to 25-50 percent)" (www.drugabuse.gov, n/p). By describing the most severe negative physical effects of addiction, NIDA, (2015), warned that heavy users suffer from "breathing illnesses, possible harm to a fetus's brain in pregnant users, and hallucinations and paranoia" (www.drugabuse.gov, n/p). In addition, Seamon, et al. (2007) reported:

Heavy marijuana use can result in psychological dysfunction, affecting a person's ability to form memories, recall events, and focus. Acute toxic psychosis induced by marijuana may be characterized by hallucinations, delusions, depersonalization (a loss of the sense of personal identity or self-recognition), fear of dying, paranoia, anxiety, changes in mood (e.g., depression), and altered mental astuteness. Marijuana has been reported to cause dose-related impairments in cognitive and behavioral functions and may impair the ability to drive a motor vehicle or operate heavy machinery. (p. 1041)

The implication was that marijuana use impacted all areas of the human experience.

**Emotional Effects**

The feelings of relaxation, the sense of deepened creativity, and improvement in perception were the attraction of using marijuana (Kuhn, et al., 2008, p.152). Continued use created an emotional attachment. As the desire for the drug increased, the frequency of use increased which then created physical dependence (Seamon, et al., 2007, p. 1039). Once an individual stopped using marijuana, withdrawal began. Symptoms of withdrawal include grouchiness, inability to sleep, loss of appetite and cravings. Anger, depression, and lethargy are common emotions that individuals experience during the withdrawal period (Kuhn, et al., p. 151-152). In the long term, as reported by NIDA (2015), "Users also report less academic and career success. For example, marijuana use is linked to a higher likelihood of dropping out of school. It is also linked to more job absences, accidents, and injuries" (www.drugabuse.gov, n/p).

**Mental Effects**

There were different types of memory dysfunction that marijuana users could suffer from. Recall there are cannabanoid receptors in the hippocampus, which involves memory function. Loss of memory and inability to focus contribute to mood swings, from anxiety to depression, while excessive use could cause acute psychosis and paranoia. (Seamon, et al., 2007, p. 1041). In addition, Kuhn, et al. (2008), found that, "In fact, the single most common and reproducible cognitive effect of marijuana is this interference with memory processing…[and that] the deficit is not in the ability to recall old, well-learned memories, but rather in the ability to form new ones" (p. 158). Without the ability to form new memories, perceptions and sense of time become distorted for the user.

## Spiritual Effects

Although marijuana had been linked to spiritual rituals throughout history, the current trends in using do not include ritual or spirituality. As reported by Bauer, Kavrakovki & Kostik (2015):

> Throughout human history marijuana has been used for many purposes such as recreation, therapy, art, religion, and medicine as a textile. The origin of marijuana dates from six thousand years ago when many different tribes used it for different celebrations and rituals. There are documents that show that marijuana was used even in the time of Chinese Emperor Shen Nung in 2337 BC. They used it in their funeral rituals. Seeds of this plant were found in their funeral urns. This plant was also used for treating insomnia, healing and also as a painkiller. Each culture and subculture from prehistory up to now use this plant because it causes selective changes in consciousness of its consumers strictly doing what is beyond reality, and also for medical reasons. (eprints.ugd.edu, n/p)

Current trends for marijuana use have been to obtain an intense and immediate high from the drug rather than having a spiritual experience. As reported by Parents Opposed To Pot (2014):

> Dabbing is inhaling the potent vapors from concentrated marijuana oil which is up to 80% THC, the psychoactive element in marijuana. In comparison, a pot cigarette contains up to 18% THC. The intense high from concentrated pot oil can literally knock you unconscious. According to

an account of a NORML event in California, one person nearly cracked their skull on the sidewalk and another experienced marijuana smoker broke her two front teeth when she passed out cold after 'dabbing'. (poppot.org, p. 2)

The intensified high intensifies the side effects. The pleasure center of the brain becomes flooded and the cannabanoid receptors become fully activated (Seamon, et al., 2007, p. 1041). Altered perception and altered sense of time contribute to a disconnection from reality. A spiritual experience was neither sought nor achieved (Seamon, et al., 2007, p. 1041).

**Effects on Sex**

Earleywine (2002) explained the sense of time slowing down described by marijuana users in this way:

> Cannabis researchers have examined cerebral blood flow (CBF) and brain metabolism, particularly in the cerebellum. This brain structure contains many cannabinoid receptors. It also plays an important role in the perception of time, which usually goes awry during cannabis intoxication. (p. 151)

Kuhn, et al. (2008), reported, "To some visual images may seem more intense or meaningful. Likewise, feelings often seem more intense for the user" (p.155). It was reasonable to assume these effects could enhance sexual experiences. Kuhn, et al. (2008), also reported that the hippocampus absorbs the THC and other chemicals, slowing breathing and motor skills. Loss of coordination during sex and

21

laborious breathing can cause fear or exasperation during intimacy and sexual intercourse (p. 150). It was reasonable to assume that these particular effects could result in an unsatisfying sexual experience.

**Stimulants**

Stimulants such as cocaine and amphetamines (Meth, Speed) increase energy in the body and brain (Friedman & Rusche, 2002, p. 110). These drugs have been used medically for weight loss, to treat attention deficit disorder and narcolepsy. As Rasmussen (2008) explained:

> Before the tough controls of the 1970s, amphetamine's main medical uses were, of course, for weight loss, depression, and a range of vaguely related psychiatric problems involving a lack of energy and efficiency. Today, the most popular medical use of speed is not so very different from this last, poorly defined category of dysfunction. The trend began with children. In the late 1930s, as we have seen, psychiatrists already knew that certain children with disruptive behavior reacted "paradoxically" to amphetamine in that they calmed down and could focus better on schoolwork. (p. 231)

Amphetamines are still used medicinally for treating ADHD and weight loss.

Another stimulant, Methylenedioxymethamphetamine (MDMA, Ecstasy, XTC), had humble beginnings as well. According to Wood and Synovitz, (2001):

MDMA, first synthesized in the early 1900s by German chemists, was patented in 1914. The earliest use of MDMA was as an appetite suppressant for soldiers during World War 1. Later, in the 1970s and early 1980s, MDMA was used therapeutically by psychotherapists to facilitate interpersonal relationships, increase self-esteem, and increase self-insight with patients. (p. 38)

The attraction for taking MDMA was its hallucinatory and euphoric qualities and its energy boost, which made it desirable for people attending rave parties (Kuhn, et al., 2008, p. 81). In the end, and to date, there are no longer any medicinal uses for MDMA (Friedman & Rusche, 2002, p. 111).

Stimulants are highly addictive and are frequently abused. As Voklow, Wang, Fowler, Thanos, Logan, Gatley, Gifford, Wong, & Pappas (2002) explained, "Studies in laboratory animals have provided evidence that dopamine (DA), a neurotransmitter involved with movement, cognition and reward, modulates predisposition to drug abuse" (p. 79). Stimulants activate the reward system in the brain. Pleasurable feelings are a natural desire in humans. As the stimulant is absorbed into the bloodstream, a physiological reaction creates a need for more pleasure. Negative consequences occur to the body, to the mind and to the spirit when trying to satisfy the need for more pleasure.

## Physical Effects

Stimulants activate the part of the brain known as the reward center. As reported by Siegel, (2013), "The brain is a collection of cells that communicate with one another using chemicals called neurotransmitters. During adolescence there is an increase in the activity of neural circuits that utilize dopamine, a central neurotransmitter central in creating our drive for reward" (p. 67). Taken recreationally and occasionally, stimulants were known to enhance social experiences, from dating to parties to sex. Athletes have been known to use stimulants for better endurance, and students have used them for better attention skills and late night studying. With the pleasure center of the brain activated, the chances for abuse are high. Siegel, (2013), continued, "All behaviors and substances that are addictive involve release of dopamine...When [it] wears off, our dopamine level plummets. We then are driven to use more of the substance that spiked our dopamine circuits" (pp. 67-68). Continuous use could cause permanent damage to the brain. According to Friedman & Rusche (2002):

> Methamphetamine has been shown to kill dopamine-containing neurons in animals, and MDMA can kill neurons that contain another neurotransmitter called serotonin. The animal data are pretty clear about this, and recent data from human MDMA abusers indicate that human users are at risk as well. (p. 110)

The constant seeking of pleasure from the dopamine depletion results in frenetic energy. As described by Kuhn, et al. (2008), "Stimulant users are in constant motion—talking, moving, exploring and generally fidgeting" (p. 231). There are many physical effects from stimulant abuse. "These include increased wakefulness, increased physical activity, decreased appetite, increased respiration, rapid heart rate, irregular heartbeat, increased blood pressure, and increased body temperature" (NIDA, 2014, www.drugabuse.gov, n/p). Cocaine abuse causes nosebleeds, headaches, seizures and death. It has been found that neurotransmitters and transmission could be permanently damaged from stimulant abuse. As Freidman & Rusche (2002) found, "There is now evidence that both people and monkeys who have self-administered cocaine for long periods of time have fewer dopamine receptors than do normal people (or monkeys, respectively)" (p. 122). Finally, MDMA has been linked to deaths at Rave concerts because of its affect to the organs. It has been reported, "Researchers have linked deaths due to MDMA overdose to the hyperthennic effect of the drug. MDMA may cause a drastic increase in core body temperature, sometimes soaring close to 110 [degrees] F, which can contribute to renal failure" (Wood & Synovitz, 2001, p. 45).

**Emotional Effects**

When describing the emotional effects of amphetamines, NIDA, (2014), reported, "Smoking or injecting the drug delivers it very quickly to the brain, where it produces an immediate, intense euphoria" (www.drugabuse.gov, n/p). Friedman & Rusche (2002) explained that,

"Although cocaine produces feelings of pleasure, it also alters perception, judgment, and thinking and has powerful effects on mood" (p. 8). The excitement and sudden burst of energy stimulants create cause users to stay awake for hours and even days at a time. The need to keep the euphoric feeling alive triggers the pleasure center. If there has been depletion of dopamine, the brain will continue to seek more pleasure. This confusion activates the sympathetic nervous system (SNS). As Kuhn, et al., (2008) related, "Epinephrine (or adrenaline) is the transmitter of the adrenal medulla, a special part of the sympathetic nervous system that is particularly important to fight-or-flight responses" (p.235). This could manifest into paranoia, hostility or violent behavior often associated with excessive stimulant abuse. (p. 235-236).

## Mental Effects

Intake of stimulants makes for an exaggerated state of joy, bursts of manufactured energy and a sense of accomplishment. Once a user stopped, the mental effects could be devastating. After coming down from their high, users experience periods of exhaustion followed by depressive symptoms such as excessive sleep and isolation (NIDA, 2014, www.drugabuse.org, n/p). According to Kuhn, et al. (2008), "One particularly difficult symptom is the inability to feel pleasure (anhedonia)" (p. 239). Anhedonia was a particularly difficult symptom to experience. "Researchers theorize that anhedonia may result from the breakdown in the brain's reward system" (Surguladze, 2003, p. 55).

This lack of pleasure created hopelessness, affecting all other aspects of a person's life.

## Spiritual Effects

Stimulants manufacture energy from the constant and repeated release of dopamine. Once using was ceased, the mind and body attempts to balance. Cravings cause anxiety and anhedonia could set in, causing an imbalance in mind/body/spirit. It was reasonable to assume that if, as Braun-Harvey (2009) stated, "Wellness is the result of improved care and balance of body, mind and spirit" (p. 25) then spiritual wellness would be difficult to achieve considering the pleasure center had been depleted and imbalance between body and mind remained.

## Effects on Sex

"Stimulants increase blood pressure and heart rate, constrict (narrow) blood vessels...and generally prepare the body for emergency...Most stimulants also increase body temperature, which presents a real problem when amphetamines are used in situations involving exercise" (Kuhn, et al., 2008, p. 232). Blood flow to sexual organs would be restricted. Without blood flow to the penis, erections would be difficult to sustain. The narrow blood vessels in the clitoris would also be restricted, making arousal and orgasm difficult. There was a possibility of death when stimulants and sex were combined. As heart rate and blood pressure increased, body temperature rose and as Kuhn (2008) explained, "...the increase in body temperature can become fatal" (p. 232). Cessation of use could result in Sexual

Anhedonia. According to Perelman (2011), "This condition means that the person will ejaculate with no accompanying sense of pleasure. The condition is most frequently found in males, but women can suffer from lack of pleasure when the body goes through the orgasm process as well" (www.sexualmed.org, n/p).

## Depressants

Opiates and Sedatives have been classified as depressants. They slow breathing, slow heart rate and relieve pain. In addition they relieve anxiety and induce sleep. In a detailed description from NIDA, (2014), the effects are as follows:

> Opioids act by attaching to specific proteins called opioid receptors, which are found in the brain, spinal cord, gastrointestinal tract, and other organs in the body. When these drugs attach to their receptors, they reduce the perception of pain. Opioids can also produce drowsiness, mental confusion, nausea, constipation, and, depending upon the amount of drug taken, can depress respiration. (www.drugabuse.gov, n/p)

The most severe side effect from opiates is death. An overdose of the drug slows the breathing "to the point that it ceases" (Kuhn, et al., 2008 p. 185).

Poppy flowers are the original source of opiates. "The oldest historic references to medicinal use of opiates arise from the Sumerian and Assyrian/Babylonian cultures (about five thousand years ago)" (Kuhn, et al, 2008, p. 186). Attractive because of its euphoric qualities, its popularity spanned centuries and continents. According to Morgan, (1982):

> In the first decades of the nineteenth century, doctors prescribed opiates widely, often merely to help the body control symptoms that no one understood, or to ease a dying patient's last hours. Opiates were seldom prescribed as an actual cure, even in an age that did not understand the causes of most diseases. They were part of a broader therapy, used chiefly to relieve distress through sedation to help nature heal the patient if the doctor's efforts failed. In a period with few sedatives, opiates were vital to the physician. Many of opium's effects were puzzling, yet the typical doctor and patient knew enough about its actions from tradition and experience to remain positive about its use. (p. 3)

The powerful pain killing effect from opiates makes them attractive for doctors (NIDA, 2014, www.drugabuse.gov, n/p). Although prescribed opiates are readily used today, tight restrictions exist for Heroin and other opiates because of their addictive qualities (Rosenberg, 2001, www.thedailybeast.com, n/p). The Comprehensive Drug Abuse Prevention and Control Act of 1970 was approved by President Nixon to classify all drugs. It was enacted to provide law enforcement and the medical community with a guideline to identify licit from illicit drugs (encyclopedia.com, 2012, n/p). The Pharmaceutical industry was given authority to regulate the drugs and required to maintain tight security and strict record keeping of their distribution.

According to Joranson (1990), concern for achieving balance in drug policy began to emerge in 1985. The primary concern was that opioids were actually being underused in the treatment of pain and in particular, cancer pain (p. 12-23). States began to create their own laws in order to gain better access to pain medications. That led to new legislation. The Prescription Drug User Fee Act of 1992 (www.fda.gov, 2012, n/p) had a major impact on drug sales. Manufacturers could now pay for approval of their product. The IMS Institute for Healthcare Formatic reported that the forecast for the "pharmerging markets" had such robust demand that annual spending on pharmaceutical medications will nearly double by 2016 (www.imshealth.com, 2013, n/p.). Newly synthesized opiates, now available in pill form, quickly became popular with dentists and pain doctors. The illusion was that because the drugs had been prescribed, they were safe to take. The addictive nature of opiates proved the opposite (Rosenberg, 2001, www.thedailybeast.com, n/p). As Girion, Glover & Smith (2011) reported, "As pain medications and OxyContin in particular became readily available more of the population became exposed to the powerful narcotic with licit drug deaths now outnumbering traffic deaths in this country" (latimes.com).

Sedatives are a class of depressants created to induce sleep. As NIDA (2014) described: "Sedatives work by slowing down brain activity resulting in drowsiness or relaxation. Many types, though, including barbiturates (like Nembutal) and benzodiazepines (like Valium and Xanax) have the potential for abuse and severe accompanying complications. At high doses or when they are abused, many of these drugs can even cause unconsciousness and death" (www.drugabuse.gov, n/p).

### Physical Effects

As explained by Friedman and Rusche, (2002), the brain is affected by opiates in this way:

> Opiates inhibit neurons, so when opiates are present, the cells fire off fewer action potentials. To keep their outputs within relatively normal limits, neurons that are constantly exposed to the inhibitory effects of opiates change other aspects of their physiology to make themselves more excitable. In essence, the changed physiology of these neurons is pulling against the way the drug is forcing them to behave. Once the drug is removed, these cells lose their balance...they then overshoot their normal level of activity and go too far in the other direction. Neurons that have been constantly inhibited by opiates become overexcited. (p. 126)

Sedatives and opiates cause drowsiness, and are used recreationally to relax, to relieve stress, and to sleep. Drooping eyes and slurred speech can be observed in a person on sedatives. Internally, the respiratory system and motor functioning in the brain slows down. Loss of memory is common. As described by Kuhn, et al., (2008), "That is, they can prevent the brain from recording and adapting to new information and changing its wiring patterns" (p. 289).

**Emotional Effects**

Euphoria comes with the initial dose of a depressant. According to Psychology Today (2014), "[Depressants] produce a relaxing effect that is beneficial to those suffering from anxiety or sleep disorders" (www.psychologytoday.com, n/p). All depressants are habit forming because tolerance builds up quickly. Higher doses are needed to get the desired effects. Anxiety levels rise as the drugs wear off. Catlin (2008) reported, "Perhaps the most insidious and cruel part of withdrawal is the depression you will most likely experience. A Depression is very common opiate withdrawal symptom and it can be quite acute" (withdrawal-ease.com, n/p).

**Mental Effects**

As reported by Friedman and Rusche, (2002), amnesia is one of the more severe side effects of depressants. Apathy, low sexual desire, and laziness are common. Catlin (2008) explained, "The depression that most people feel is centered around the guilt and shame of their predicament. Many people have feelings of worthlessness and dread as well as feelings that their situation will never get better" (withdrawal-ease.com, n/p).

**Spiritual Effects**

Depression contributes to spiritual illness. Negative feelings like shame and guilt contribute to spiritual illness (Wesselman and Kuykendall, 2004, p. 74). One symptom of spiritual illness is called disharmony. Wesselman, et al., (2004), stated, "Disharmony is what we experience when life suddenly loses its meaning or when we have lost an important connection to life" (p. 75). When an addict quits using, the fear of being disconnected can be overwhelming. Well-being can be compromised when using opiates and sedatives. Depressants cause physiological disconnections from body and mind. Additionally, "The most dangerous thing about the opiate drug, by far – and the usual cause of death – is the suppression of breathing" (Kuhn, et al., 2008, p. 199). As the respiratory system slows down, less oxygen flows through the brain, and according to Kuhn, et al., (2008), causes the individual "to become sedated and sleepy" (p. 199). As explained by Wesselman, et al., (2004):

> The state of disharmony that we experience in response to such life situations causes a diminishment of our personal power. This can happen in a subtle manner on the one hand, or in a catastrophic, life-shaking way on the other like losing your job, and in the process losing your livelihood. When we experience disempowerment, or "power loss," it affects our energetic matrix, rendering us vulnerable to illness. (p. 76)

That power loss, or powerlessness, has been considered the point of realization for an addict and alcoholic. It could lead to recovery.

### Effects on Sex

Sex is difficult for a person using depressants. Difficulties remained when the person stopped using them. Caitlin (2008) described it in this way:

33

> If you're addicted to pain killers, they not only hamper your physical ability to "perform" they also probably lessen your libido. One of the only not-so-unpleasant side effects of opiate withdrawal that you may notice -if you decide to quit- is that you become extremely amorous. Extremely. I was in no condition to actually have sex during my Vicodin withdrawals but it's amazing how much these pills hamper your desire to do the absolute best thing in the world. (withdrawal-ease.com, n/p)

It was reasonable to conclude that having sex while using depressants would be possible but not desired. Conversely, once a person quit using depressants, desire returned but the ability to perform did not (Caitlin, 2008, withdrawal-ease.com, n/p).

## Alcohol

According to Kuhn, et al., (2008), alcohol was the most accessible drug available. It did not need a prescription, and it was sold over the counter (p. 36). Considered a sedative hypnotic, it was classified unto its own rather, than as a depressant because of its biphasic quality. As described by Kuhn, et al, (2008), "This [biphasic quality] refers to the fact that at low concentrations alcohol actually activates some nerve cells. As the alcohol concentration increases, however, these same cells decrease their firing rates and their activities become depressed" (p. 41).

Alcohol consumption is desired for its euphoric qualities (Alcoholics Anonymous, 1952, p. xxvi). Its effects depend on two things: body size and the amount taken into the body. Drink sizes are measured in ounces (The National Institute on Alcohol Abuse and

Alcoholism (NIAAA), 2010, p.4). According to NIAAA one standard drink equals 12 ounces of beer, 8 to 9 fluid ounces of malt liquor, 5 fluid ounces of table wine and 1.5 fluid ounces of 80-proof distilled spirits" (p. 4). The Office of Alcohol and Drug Education (OADE) (2015) explained, "The less you weigh, the more you will be affected by a given amount of alcohol. For people of the same weight, even the same gender, individuals with a lower percentage of body fat will have lower BAC's than those with a higher percentage of body fat" (oade.nd.edu, n/p.) Being fat soluble, women could feel the effects from drinking more quickly than men and could suffer physical consequences more quickly. In addition, as reported by OADE (2015):

> Women have less of the enzyme dehydrogenase that breaks down alcohol in the stomach contributing to higher BAC's than men drinking the same amount of alcohol. Hormone levels also affect the body's ability to process alcohol, and women will experience higher BAC's drinking their regular amount of alcohol right before menstruation. Women tend to have a higher percentage of body fat and a lower percentage of water. (oade.nd.edu, n/p.)

Judgment, motor skills, body temperature and organs are all negatively affected by alcohol (NIAAA, 2010, p.5)

**Physical Effects**

Alcohols effect on the body is widespread, and begins with the central nervous system (CNS). Pietrangelo (2014) described the action in this way:

One of the first signs of alcohol in your system is a change in behavior. Alcohol travels through the body easily. It can quickly reach many parts of your body, including your brain and other parts of your central nervous system. That can make it harder to talk, causing slurred speech, the telltale sign that someone has had too much to drink. It can also affect coordination, interfering with balance and the ability to walk. (www.healthline.com, n/p)

The list continued with all major systems being affected (excretory, digestive, circulatory, skeletal, muscular and immune) as well as sexual and reproductive health (Pietrangello, 2014, www.healthline.com, n/p).

The effects on the brain are many. Dopamine activity begins as alcohol levels rise in the bloodstream, causing a rush. Once the alcohol levels out in the bloodstream, the dopamine neurons stop activating. Extended and excessive use could cause permanent damage to the brain as explained by Harper (1998):

There is brain shrinkage in uncomplicated alcoholics, which can largely be accounted for by loss of white matter. Some of this damage appears to be reversible. However, alcohol-related neuronal loss has been documented in specific regions of the cerebral cortex (superior frontal association cortex), hypothalamus (supraoptic and paraventricular nuclei), and cerebellum. (journals.lww.com, n/p)

Harper's findings revealed that brain shrinkage takes place in the executive functioning part of the brain, the frontal cortex, which controls motor skills and memory. Wernicke-Korsakoff syndrome, or wet brain, is one of the most severe effects on the brain from alcohol abuse. The symptoms of Wernicke encephalopathy and Kosakoff psychosis occur due to Vitamin B1 deficiency. As explained by the U. S. National Library of Medicine (2015):

> Wernicke encephalopathy and Korsakoff syndrome are different conditions. Both are due to brain damage caused by a lack of vitamin B1...Lack of vitamin B1 is common in people with alcoholism...Korsakoff syndrome, or Korsakoff psychosis, tends to develop as Wernicke symptoms go away. Wernicke encephalopathy causes brain damage in lower parts of the brain called the thalamus and hypothalamus. Korsakoff psychosis results from permanent damage to areas of the brain involved with memory. Some symptoms, especially the loss of memory and thinking skills, may be permanent. Other disorders related to alcohol use may also occur. (www.nlm.nih.gov, n/p)

Cirrhosis of the Liver, dehydration, malnutrition, heart attacks, strokes, and cancer in the esophagus were some of the more severe physical side effects from alcohol consumption (OADE, 2015, oade.nd.edu, n/p.).

**Emotional Effects**

The biphasic quality of alcohol contributes to alcohol's emotional effects (Kuhn, et al., 2008, p. 32). The stimulating buzz from the first drink activates the pleasure center in the brain. According to Roland (2010):

Once it begins circulating in the body, it decreases activity within the nervous system. When you drink alcohol, you may notice that you have more feelings of depression or that you become stuck in a state of depression as a result of drinking. In addition, as you consume large amounts of alcohol, you may become stressed from the impact of the drug. While the buzz from alcohol can initially be enjoyable, it can give way to a series of stresses on the system that will manifest psychologically. Alcohol use can result in restlessness, nightmares, and even overwhelming fear. (www.med.upenn.edu, n/p)

## Mental Effects

Personality is affected by alcohol as well as moods. As Roland (2010) found:

More generally, excessive alcohol use can lead to personality changes. Your usual interaction style can be altered drastically by an intoxicating amount of alcohol. You may become selfish, egotistical, or even susceptible to mood swings and aggressive behavior. These changes are brought on by the effects of alcohol on serotonin in your body. Serotonin is a neurotransmitter in your body that transmits signals related to mood. When the effect of serotonin is weakened by an excess of alcohol, chemical imbalances result in aggressive behavior or mood swings. (www.med.upenn.edu, n/p)

Aggression has been linked to alcohol, but so has subservience. As reported by Anderson, Spruille, Venable, & Strano (2005), "Males were more likely to take advantage of someone sexually and to be taken advantage of sexually after heavy episodic drinking. In contrast, females were more likely to be taken advantage of by someone sexually but not more likely to take advantage of someone sexually after heavy episodic drinking" (www.ejhs.org). It was reasonable to conclude that people are more likely to act impulsively when inebriated, resulting in behaviors they would not normally engage in while sober.

**Spiritual Effects**

U. S. National Library of Medicine, 2015, stated that the adoration of alcohol makes it difficult to for people to understand the true nature of alcohol: toxic and addicting (www.nlm.nih.gov, n/p). The Social Issues Research Centre (SIRC), (2014), contended:

> At the simplest level, drinks are used to define the nature of the occasion. In many Western cultures, for example, champagne is synonymous with celebration, such that if champagne is ordered or served at an otherwise 'ordinary' occasion, someone will invariably ask "What are we celebrating?" (p. 25)

In addition, the spiritual aspect of alcohol in religious ceremonies gave credence to its use. As asserted by Phillips (2014), "The relationship between alcohol and religion began thousands of years ago" (p. 45). The feeling it produced was a much sought-after feeling and it belied its dangers. A doctor who worked with alcoholics in the

1930's wrote in Alcoholics Anonymous (1955), "Men and women drink essentially because they like the effect produced by alcohol (p. xxvi). The doctor described the feeling as so elusive people consume more and more to find it. The repeated search for that elusive feeling brings dependence. One synonym for alcohol was "spirits" (www.thesaurus.com, n/p). Spirit was sought from a bottle rather than from within the soul.

**Effects on Sex**

True connection with another person is difficult when inebriated (Shuster, 1988, p. 2). As previously reported, personality changes occur due to chemical imbalance in the brain (www.med.upenn.edu, n/p). The effects include poor judgment and risky behavior (Pietrangello, 2014, www.healthline.com, n/p).

There is a common belief that alcohol and sex go together well, taking away inhibitions and giving libido a boost, (Shuster, 1988, p. 63). From his research, which examined the effects of alcohol consumption on female sexuality, Shuster (1988) determined that belief to be false:

> It was found that women's beliefs about the aphrodisiac properties of alcohol did not correspond to daily logs of sexual and drinking activity. The women thought that alcohol enhanced their sexual desire and increased their activity and enjoyment. The logs reflected the reverse. Alcohol consumption was correlated with decreased initiation of sexual activity by the subjects. (p. 65)

Additional research on female sexuality by Shuster (1988), "indicated a progressive decrease in vaginal engorgement and an increase in orgasmic latency with increasing blood alcohol concentrations" (p. 71). His results suggested that women were left without desire for sex and without enjoyment during sex when consuming alcohol (Shuster, 1988, p. 71).

For men, Shuster (1988) reported, "Although alcohol in low doses has been thought to have a disinhibiting effect, leading to promiscuity or, at least, diminished shyness in making sexual overtures, decrease in frequency of intercourse has been ascribed to heavy drinking" (p. 2). Infrequency of intercourse put strains on intimate relationships. Shuster continued, "Alcohol increases libido in small doses because of its disinhibiting and anxiety-reducing effect on higher cortical centers. However, in high doses it is found to produce impotence" (p. 2). The results were equally disturbing for men, for alcohol consumption left them with less desire and possible inability to have sexual intercourse (Shuster, 1988, p. 2).

Levine (2007) asserted, "The Buddha saw sexual energy as the strongest of all energies in existence, and perhaps the most difficult to relate to skillfully" (p. 83). Since alcohol affected every system and every organ in the body (NIAAA, 2010, p. 2-20) the skill to relate to sexuality was difficult to achieve.

## Conclusions about Mind-Altering Substances

Mind-altering substances were not necessarily a problem for many individuals, and in fact were often included in cultural celebrations and of maturity or adulthood (Siegel, 2013, p. 7). It has been found that many people have used mind-altering substances to enhance certain life events, forge relationships with others and to have sex. Marijuana has been found to effect perception, and cause apathy (Kuhn, et al., 2008, p. 150). Stimulants were shown to manufacture energy and, if abused, deplete neurotransmitters in the pleasure center of the brain resulting in anhedonia, the inability to feel pleasure (Kuhn, et al., 2008, p. 239). Depressants have been used to ease pain, calm anxiety, and slow breathing. They also create rising body temperatures, which could lead to death during physical exertion, including sex (NIDA, 2014, www.drugabuse.gov, n/p). Alcohol was found to cause disinhibition, which could lead to heightened desire for intimacy and sex. It was also found to contribute to unhealthy sexual practices, aggressive behaviors and inability to reach orgasm in both men and women (Shuster, 1988, p. 71). Many substances were found to be addictive. Negative consequences to the body, including the brain, mind and spirit created difficulties in having sex. The road to recovery included rebuilding the brain, rediscovering the body, reconnecting with the mind, and recreating sexual ideals in order to have enjoyable sex in sobriety (Levine, 2007, p. 83).

## Mindfulness Practices

The information for this study was derived from literature with historical and current perspectives and from the scientific community. An historic background from the teachings of the Buddha, to Modern Era Mindfulness Practitioners and Teachers, including but not limited to authors Noah Levine, and Jack Kornfield were explored. Other information was derived from articles published for various websites that included the American Medical Association, The Center for Mindfulness and The Omega Institute for Holistic Studies. In addition, Anne Cushman, and Chip Hartranet were among the authors reviewed for Mindful Yoga practices.

"The practice of Mindfulness starts simply by cultivating the capacity to be alert to the body, most of the time, except during sleep. This process begins with the capability to be aware what we hear, see, sense, touch and taste and whether these are pleasant, unpleasant or neutral" (Biddulph & Flynn, 2009, p.143). Cultivating awareness takes time and care. Mindfulness is an ongoing and active endeavor. Germer (2009) described it to be like planting a garden: Cultivation of the mind was like planting the seeds of awareness, shining light into the garden of the spirit and allowing time for growth (p. 46). This was called Mindfulness. Mindfulness was an alternate and holistic means of affecting the mind and the body rather than using mind-altering substances (Kabat-Zinn, 1996, p. x). Meditation and yoga were the tools to be used to cultivate that alertness (Levine, 2007, p. 130).

Mindfulness brings awareness to the body, mind and spirit. Understanding the Four Foundations of Mindfulness: body, feelings, mind and mental qualities, is the first step in practicing Mindfulness. As translated by Bhikkhu (2008), "There is the case where a monk remains focused on the body in & of itself — ardent, alert, & Mindful — putting aside greed & distress with reference to the world. He remains focused on feelings... mind... mental qualities in & of themselves — ardent, alert, & Mindful — putting aside greed & distress with reference to the world" (p. MN10).

The inception of Mindfulness dates back some 2000 years ago. Biddulph & Flynn (2009) reported that "Although there is little dispute that Siddhartha actually existed, accounts of his life are a blend of historical fact and legend" (p. 18). According to Biddulph, et al., (2009), "Prince Siddhartha Gautama...was born between 563 and 483 BCE" (p. 18). The authors then described the story of his childhood; that his mother had died just days after his birth, and that his father kept him sheltered in the Palace to protect him. They recalled the legend of Prince Siddhartha being that he became disturbed during a day outside. He witnessed things he had never seen before: "an old man, a sick man, a corpse" (p.19). His Gentleman servant explained the suffering of each one to him. The Prince then witnessed another man wandering around the streets in a robe. He was told that the man in the robe was a spiritual leader, dedicated to finding the meaning of life and death. Returning to the Palace, The Prince remained unsettled by the suffering he had witnessed. In concluding, Biddulph, et al., (2009), explained, "These 'four sights' are said to have been what finally prompted the prince to question his life and embark on a spiritual quest" (p. 19). After many days and nights of seeking, as he sat in meditation under a tree, he became enlightened with the wisdom that the way to end suffering came from power within. Self-awareness was the way to end suffering. He called himself Buddha, and taught his newfound wisdom until he died. (p. 21-23)

Meditation and yoga have been familiar topics in the U. S. for decades. Mindfulness has been linked with the field of Psychology (Germer, 2009, p. 4), Stress Reduction Clinics (Kabat-Zinn, 1990, p. 9) and Modern Buddhist practices (Levine, 2007, p. 13). Currently, science has found a way to actually measure its benefits using imaging technology. As reported by Holzel, Carmody, Congleton, & Yerramsetti (2011), a virtual photograph of the brain could be taken, which could provide a visual recording of brain activity, and was used to measure the effects of Mindfulness practices on the brain. "Neuroimaging studies have begun to explore the neural mechanisms underlying Mindfulness meditation practice with techniques such as electroencephalography (EEG) and functional magnetic resonance imaging (MRI)" (p. 36).

Mindfulness' acceptance into the Medical Community began when Jon Kabat-Zinn (1990) created Mindfulness Based Stress Reduction (MBSR). Patients suffering from chronic pain considered beyond any more hope were sent to his stress clinic. Being a practicing Buddhist he understood that suffering came from within. He was able to use his experience to help others. His message was about self-empowerment over suffering explaining, "All of us have the capacity to be Mindful. All it involves is cultivating our ability to pay attention in the present moment" (p. 9-11). His philosophy was that of learning how to work with what you have, including chronic physical pain, asserting, "In such cases the quality of your life may greatly depend on your own ability to know your body and mind well enough to work at optimizing your own health within bounds, always unknown, of what may be possible" (p. 27). Germer (2009) elaborated on the importance of Mindful awareness when facing emotional pain, stating, "Difficult emotions become destructive and break down the mind, body and spirit...Usually we're not aware just how many of these trials have their root in how we relate to the inevitable discomfort of life" (p. 2). Mindfulness is used to create a new way of relating to those "inevitable discomforts of life" (p. 2). Currently, Mindfulness practices have been integrated into modern psychotherapy. Germer (2009) explained:

Mindfulness is considered an underlying factor in effective psychotherapy and emotional healing in general. When therapy goes well, patients (or clients) develop an accepting attitude toward whatever they're experiencing in the therapy room—fear, anger, sadness, joy, relief, boredom, love—and this benevolent attitude gets transferred to daily life. A special bonus of Mindfulness is that it can be practiced at home in the form of meditation. (p. 4)

## Meditation

Meditation, as defined by Merriam-Webster (2015), is "to engage in mental exercise (as concentration on one's breathing or repetition of a mantra) for the purpose of reaching a heightened level of spiritual awareness" (www.merriam-webster.com, n/p). There are two forms of meditation practice: *"formal"* referring to setting a regular time and place to cultivate awareness, and *"informal"* referring to bringing awareness into all aspects of daily life (Kabat-Zinn, 1996, p. 2). As described by Levine, (2007), "The formal training of Mindfulness takes place on the meditation cushion, through redirecting the attention or awareness to the breath, body, feeling tone and process of the mind, as well as the state of mind that has arisen" (p. 42). Formal practice is the foundation of Mindfulness. The body is the foundation of Mindfulness training.

**Body**

Since formal practice takes place in a form of the lotus position, sitting on a cushion with legs crossed, it is necessary to direct attention to its effect on the body. Sitting for an extended period of time on a cushion, with crossed legs and an erect spine, could be painful. The legs could fall asleep, the lower back could begin to spasm, and ankles and feet could go numb. It takes practice. The position has not varied much for 2000 years. Cushman (2014) addressed the history of the lotus position and its importance in this way:

> In ancient India, chairs didn't exist: Everyone sat cross-legged on the ground or on low cushions, and so from early childhood, their hips and lower backs adapted to that position...What is important, if you're going to do formal meditation practice for any length of time, is the alignment of your head, neck, spine and pelvis. A spine that's balanced and at ease supports the relaxation of your whole nervous system. (p. 118)

Once in a seated and balanced position with the whole nervous system beginning to relax, the breath becomes the initial focus of meditation. Breathing is automatic and familiar, which makes it a comfortable place to begin. As explained by Germer (2009),

"Mindfulness of breath cultivates focus on a single object, but you shouldn't expect your attention to remain unwaveringly with the breath. Just return your attention again and again to the breath when you notice your mind wander" (p. 46). With attention given to the breath, a thought, memory, or idea may enter the mind. It was to be noticed and then attention to be returned to the breath. The act of returning again and again from the wandering mind to the breath is the training needed for present-time awareness. Levine (2007) related, "This natural process of training the mind is the essence of meditation. It is important to understand that this will happen over and over. Bring the attention back to the simple experience of the breath over and over" (p. 130).

The next step is to expand the field of awareness from the breath to the body. Germer (2009) asserted, "We shouldn't think that the body is less important than the mind when practicing Mindfulness...since the body is relatively slow and stable, it's an excellent vantage point for observing our mind and emotions." (P. 49).

Levine (2007) advised that after about ten minutes of focusing on the breath, attention could be brought to the whole body. Attention is brought to the sensation of the pressure of the pelvis on the cushion, and the contact points of hands and fingers on the legs. As the mind wanders into thoughts and emotions, they are noticed and then the attention is brought back to the breath. Once connection with the breath is reestablished, expanded awareness could go back to the body. This directing and redirecting of attention is building a foundation to work from; present-time awareness could then come more easily (p.

131-132). Levine (2007) continued, "With the foundation of present-time awareness, as established by the continual returning of the attention to the breath and body, you can now allow the attention to expand to include all of the sense doors" directing attention to sounds, smells and even sights. (p. 132).

Meditation affects the brain in a variety of ways. When considering that sitting meditation brings relaxation to the whole nervous system, (Cushman, 2014, p. 118), Hanson & Mendius (2009) explained, "If you want to use your mind-body connection to lower your stress, cool your fires, and improve your long-term health, what's the optimal point of entry? It's the autonomic nervous system (ANS)" (p. 80). Signals are sent from the ANS to the brain. The brain responds, first in the sympathetic nervous system (SNS), triggering fight-or flight and second, the parasympathetic nervous system (PNS). Hanson, et al. (2009), continued:

> The PNS conserves energy in your body and is responsible for ongoing, steady-state activity. It produces a feeling of relaxation often with a sense of contentment—this is why it's sometimes called the 'rest-and-digest' system, in contrast to the 'fight-or-flight' SNS. (p. 59)

The PNS calms the SNS, and in turn the brain, signals the muscles to relax and signals the breath to remain normal.

Further research suggested that meditation increases gray matter in the brain (Holzel, et al., 2011, p. 36). Technology has enabled the scientific community to peer into the brain. Neuroimaging is being used to see if meditation not only provides psychological changes, but physical changes to the brain as well. Images of the brain have shown gray matter increases in the hippocampus and right interior insula after a period of practicing Mindful meditation. Holzel, et al. (2011), explained:

> The hippocampus is known to be critically involved in learning and memory processes and in the modulation of emotional control while the insula has been postulated to play a key role in the process of awareness – functions which have been shown to be important in the process and outcomes of Mindfulness training. (p. 36-37)

In addition, "A growing body of literature has demonstrated that neural systems are modifiable networks and changes in neural structure can occur in adults as a result of training" (Draganski, Gaser, Busch, Schuierer, Bogdahn & May, 2004, p. 38). The importance of these findings seems crucial for people in recovery as they lend credence to the possibility that meditation could repair parts of the brain that were negatively affected by substance abuse.

Addiction involves intense desire for stimulation, for pleasure. Meditation could be used to stimulate the brain in similar fashion. Hanson, et al. (2009), described specific methods to increase stimulation during meditation that had proven to be useful for those with a "spirited temperament" (p. 197) and they included:

- Noticing individual qualities of the breath. Draw in new information, paying attention to details, such as the sensations at different spots on the upper lip.

- Focus on multiple sensations in a large area of your body such as the chest. Or notice how breathing creates sensations all over your body, such as subtle movements in your hips and head.

- Do walking meditation, which provides more stimulation than sitting quietly. (p.197)

**Feelings**

Levine (2007) explained when practicing Mindfulness, tones of feelings are to be observed. Feeling tones are not emotions. Feeling tones require that attention be paid to whether an experience is pleasant, unpleasant, or neutral. Pleasant feelings come from being satisfied with an experience. Unpleasant feelings signify disturbance from emotional or physical pain and resisting the unpleasant feeling. Neutral tones are just that. The feeling tone of neutrality is neither pleasant nor unpleasant. Attention to feeling tones is the way to arrive into present-time awareness (p. 133-134). Levine (2007) continued:

> While sitting with awareness focused on the body, refine the attention to the feeling tone of your experience. Investigate and inquire into the nature of the experience you are paying attention to. Is this a pleasant feeling? Does it feel good? Or is it an uncomfortable experience? Are you resisting the present feeling? Bring Mindfulness to the feeling itself; see how you relate to pleasure and pain. (p. 134)

Accessing a neutral tone creates an opportunity to investigate the mind's need to seek pleasure or pain. Continued training of the mind helps uncover attachments to all things pleasurable and to those that brought pain. The awareness practices aid in identification of those thoughts, noticing craving or aversion, and then setting them aside to live in present-time awareness. Hanson, et al. (2009), reasoned, "If you can break the link between feeling tones and craving—if you can be with the pleasant without chasing after it, with the unpleasant without resisting it, and the neutral without ignoring it—then you have cut the chain of suffering" (p. 113-114).

Establishing awareness of feeling tones, learning how to experience pleasant, unpleasant and neutral phenomena as they come and go was, as Levine (2007) described, "...the key on the meditative path" (p. 135).

**Mind**

Cultivating awareness of the mind is the next step on the meditative path. According to Levine (2007), the thinking mind has two parts: process and content. It is important to meditate on the process separate from its content. He explained:

> Meditate on the mind as a process. Each thought is like a bubble floating through the spaciousness of awareness. One may contain a plan, another a memory, and yet another a judgment or emotion. Allow each thought to pass without getting into the bubble or floating off with it. Until meditation practice is matured, you will get seduced by the thinking mind over and over...As with the breath,

simply let go and return to the present over and over, bursting the bubble and redirecting attention to the process again and again. (p. 135-136)

Meditation directed the mind to pay attention to this process, which eventually transformed the relationship one had to the contents. After establishing awareness of thoughts arising and passing, the mind could then be directed towards the content of each mind-moment. Levine (2007) described content of the mind in this way:

After expanding the attention to the process of the thinking mind and observing the passing of thoughts, bring attention to the contents of each mind-moment. Know directly the truth of each thought. Be aware of the memory as a memory, and when a plan arises in the mind know it as a plan. (p. 136-137)

Meditation helps the mind continue to process thoughts, and Mindfulness continues to identify the truth of its content. As Hay (2004) explained, "Thoughts have no power over us unless we give in to them. Thoughts are only words strung together. They have NO MEANING WHATSOEVER. Only *we* give meaning to them. Let us choose to think thoughts that nourish and support us" (p. 79). Mindfulness helps one to make a choice. Meditation supports a deliberate change in the thought processes of people in recovery.

## Mental Qualities

In Mindfulness, mental qualities are the emotional state of the mind and spirit (Kornfield, 2008, p. 55). Having learned how to attend to breathing, thoughts, feeling tone, present-time awareness and mind-moment it was now possible to focus on the emotional state attached to them. Through meditation, deliberate intention towards positive emotions would replace negative emotions. Mindfulness practices provide the ability to notice the true nature of the mind. As Kornfield (2008) related:

> When we look at our own mind, we can notice the mental states that predominate, as if we were noticing the weather. Just as a storm can bring rain, wind, and cold, we can observe the clusters of unhealthy states that appear on our bad days. We may find resentment, fear, anger, worry, doubt, envy or agitation. We can notice how often they arise and how attached we are to their point of view. We can also notice healthy states in our most free and openhearted periods. We can notice how love, generosity, flexibility, ease and simplicity are natural to us. They give us trust in our goodness, our own Buddha nature. (p. 56-57)

Healthy states of mind are available through metta meditation. "*Metta* is a Pali word that is generally translated as 'love' or, more often 'loving-kindness'" (Cushman, 2014, p. 154). Metta-meditation phrases add compassionate intention to formal meditation. Uttered in silence or out loud, repeated messages of love and kindness were to be directed towards self and towards others. In the words of Kornfield

(2008), metta assists in cultivating "love, generosity, flexibility, ease and simplicity" (p. 57).

As outlined by Hanson, et al. (2009), after settling into formal practice, breathing normally with a relaxed body, an intention was to be set to direct love and kindness to an object. The intention was metta, or loving-kindness, and it was directed to the self first. Phrases that contained wishes of safety, happiness, ease, and comfort were repeated as often as desired. Then they were to be directed outward, wishing for others to receive the same messages of compassion, and repeating them as often as desired. The intention of loving-kindness was to be incorporated into daily life as the practice deepened (p. 159-160). The authors suggested, "Throughout the day, deliberately bring kindness into your actions, your speech and most of all your thoughts...Try experiments in which you bring loving-kindness to someone for a specific period of time—perhaps a family member for an evening, or a coworker during a meeting—and see what happens. Also act kindly to yourself—and see what that's like!" (p. 160).

At the Center for Mindfulness in Medicine, Healthcare and Society, studies showed physical changes to the part of the brain linked to emotions after participation in an 8-week Mindfulness Based Stress Reduction program. Carmody & Baer (2008) reported, "Participation in the Mindfulness Based Stress Reduction (MBSR) program appears to be associated with improvements in trait (genetically determined characteristics) and state (learned characteristics) psychological distress and medical symptoms" (p. 2). Scientific evidence supported the theory that Mindfulness meditation was responsible for increased gray matter concentration in the hippocampus, and for improving the ability to regulate emotions (Carmody & Baer, 2008, p. 2). Research done by Luders, (2010), at The UCLA Lab of Neuroimaging, found similar results. She reported, "Because these areas of the brain are so closely linked to emotion, these might be the neuronal underpinnings that give meditators the outstanding ability to regulate their emotions and allow for well-adjusted responses to whatever life throws their way" (www.sciencedaily.com, n/p).

Whole brain images revealed grey matter growth in the region of the brain that regulates emotions. A study conducted by Holzel, et al. (2011), revealed growth in the hippocampal region of the brain. The images came from MRI's of an MBSR sample group and a control group. The neuroimaging took place two weeks prior to participation in an 8-week MBSR program (pre-test) and two weeks after the 8-week MBSR program was completed (post-test). The images showed increases in gray matter in the MBSR group, but not the control group. Whole brain analysis also revealed greater concentration of gray matter at the time of post-test in the MBSR group as compared with gray matter concentration at the time of pre-test in the MBSR group. The two regions that showed increases of gray matter were the posterior cingulate cortex (PCC) and the left temporoparietal junction (TPJ) (p. 42). They submitted their findings as "...suggesting that participation in an MBSR course causes structural changes in these regions" (Holzel, et al., 2011, p. 42). It was reasonable to assume that growth in that region of the brain could affect change in emotions.

**Effects on Sex Life**

The awareness gained through meditation can be applied to sex. A mind previously occupied by drugs and alcohol was now in need of finding new ways to generate pleasure. As Levine (2007) elucidated, the Buddha viewed sexual desire as being the strongest of all desires. He asserted, "Not just the act of sex, but the whole realm of sexuality, including intimacy, procreation, sexual pleasure and loving relationships" (p. 83).

Braun-Harvey (2009) counseled people in recovery about the difficulties of sober sex. He emphasized:

- Recovery is a process of learning how to have intense emotional feelings and manage these feelings without resorting to drugs and alcohol.

- Anyone who is committed to sobriety and recovery is going to have a wide variety of feelings that may at the time seem unmanageable.

- Feelings of attractions, desire, having a crush, lusting for someone, or having love dreams are all part of life and part of recovery.

- What protects a person in recovery from destructive behavior in coping with unmanageable feelings is talking about them in a safe and non-shaming place.

- As we will see in our recovery skills for relationship and marriage, focusing on yourself and developing who you are as a person is a much more important focus. (p. 84)

The process of focusing on self and learning how to manage intense emotions involved Mindfulness and meditation. The road to enjoyable sex in recovery included paying attention to negative emotions attached to sex. Levine (2007) maintained:

The issue here is not sexual energy itself, then, since that's an innately human characteristic. The difficulty we face lies in our inner relationship of attachment to pleasure. On the cushion in meditation practice, we begin to understand that clinging, attachment, and aversion are the primary causes of the extra layer of suffering that we create for ourselves. We begin to see, through paying attention to the breath, body, emotions, and mind, that if we allow everything that arises to pass, we will experience a quality of satisfaction in pure awareness, in the natural arising and passing away of our mind states and sensations. (p. 85)

Bringing compassion to sexual energy creates a new a way to manage the intense negative emotions that have been unmanageable for someone in recovery. By focusing on breathing and incorporating positive feelings in meditation, emotional shifts begin to emerge.

The first shifts begin in the brain. As Hanson, et al. (2009), reported, deliberate concentration on *sensations* of breathing activate the regions of the brain that support working memory. The regions of the brain remain stable until information passes through (p. 179). They describe a kind of gate that protects the working memory from other information coursing through the brain. "When the gate is closed, you stay focused on one thing. When a new stimulus comes knocking—or sound of a bird—the gate pops open allowing new information in to update working memory" (p. 179).

Directing positive intention into the mind causes a shift towards a healthy emotional state (Kornfield, 2009, p. 57). As suggested by Hanson, et al. (2009), there are two strong intentions that could elevate mood: rapture and joy. The authors continued, "Positive feelings help concentrate attention by causing steadily high transmission of dopamine to the neural substrate of working memory...Thus, the more enjoyable and intense your feelings are, the greater the dopamine release—and the more concentrated your attention" (p. 198). They encouraged integrating rapture and joy with the breath and making *them* the object of the intention. The reason for making rapture and joy the objects of intention, according to Hanson, et al (2009), was to "Get a clear sense of each state so you can call it to mind in the future" (p. 199). The ability to call upon rapture and joy to the mind at a future point in time is a useful tool for regulating emotions. As reported by Kettlehack (1993), sober sex could be frightening (p. 3). Calling forth rapture and joy just before sex was a practical solution for those in recovery whose sober sex experiences had been filled with fear and would like to experience enjoyable sober sex.

Situated next to the hippocampus is the amygdala. Salu (2013) reported that the function of the amygdala is to respond to emotionally charged stimuli. As reported by Hanson et al. (2009), the SNS and PNS activate fight-or-flight and safety signals. When the amygdala receives emotionally charged stimuli, it then records its findings, creating an emotional attachment to the memory. As Salu (2013) explained:

The amygdala is an important brain center that handles various aspects of fear and safety. It is involved in learning new cues, in creating memory records, and in supporting information retrieval in other processes. The [research] suggests that the amygdala is involved in sexual-arousal through its handling of fear and safety information. Another tenet of the [research], which is corroborated by experimental findings, is that the information structures that support sexual-arousal are built by conditioning. The [research] illustrates how conditioning of non-sexual experiences creates the cues for sexual-arousal. (www.ejhs.org, n/p.)

Salu (2013) found sexual arousal to be a conditioned response from non-sexual experiences (www.ejhs.org, n/p.). Since the use of drugs and alcohol also affected the amygdala, it was possible the conditioned responses for sexual-arousal were distorted, false or missing. Conditioned responses for sexual-arousal needed to be reconditioned (Salu, 2013, www.ejhs.org, n/p). Mindfulness practices facilitated reconditioning of those responses (Levine, 2007, p. 91).

According to Levine (2007), "When we practice Mindfulness and allow sexual energy to be the object of awareness, rather than allowing ourselves to be a slave to the libido's ever request, we begin to relate *to* sexuality rather than *from* it" (p. 91). Reconditioning of sexual-arousal responses in the brain, and paying attention becomes easier with practice. He continued, "When sexuality is related to skillfully, it becomes our teacher rather than our tormentor. It becomes just another experience in the mind and body that we can and should pay close attention to" (Levine, 2007, p. 91).

Sex in recovery becomes a different experience. Continued practice of Mindful meditation, provides an ability to change the mind-state of fear into joy and rapture. It facilitates the ability to bring present-time awareness to the sexual experience. Sensations feel more intense because there are no more distractions from mind-altering substances. The feeling tones of pleasant, unpleasant and neutral could now come into focus.. Enjoyable sober sex could now possible (Levine, 2007, p. 95).

## Yoga

The ancient translation for yoga was "yoking" or "union" (Hartranet, 2003, p. 133), bringing body and breath together. The modern translation is, as described by Cushman (2014), "The art of transforming consciousness by directly working with physical form—enlivening the physical body while liberating the heart and mind" (p. xvi). Yoga unites the body, the breath and the mind.

Hartranet (2003) described an Eight Fold Yogic Path that integrates the body, mind, and spirit as a whole. He explained, "With the word *yoga*, Patañjali is describing a process of interiorization that begins with one's relation to externals, then to self, body, breath, orientation of attention, focus, absorption, and finally merger" (p. 31). Translated by Lord (2011), "The Sutras break yoga down into 8 limbs which include asanas (physical yoga poses), meditation and something called *yamas*. The yamas are 5 ethical teachings dealing with how we relate to the external world" (spiritvoyage.com, n/p). She listed the 5 ethical principles as being non-violence, truthfulness, non-stealing, non-excess, and non-greediness. The body, mind and spirit are affected by external forces, which included environment, interpersonal relationships, diet and exercise, familial values, culture, social status, appearance, successes and failures. Identification of the external forces is the key to awareness. The awareness of emotional attachment to the external forces leads to understanding. Understanding illuminates how we relate to the attachments and yamas are to be practiced to open space and affect change.

Recovery was the beginning of change for an individual. Many individuals in recovery have been neglecting their bodies and minds for years (Alcoholics Anonymous, 1952, p. 157). Yoga provides a gentle return to one's body and mind. The intention during yoga is simple; pay attention to the breath and the body.

**Body**

The first yoga asana, or pose is to be neutral: sitting, standing, or lying down. Noticing the breath, attention is to focus on sensations in the body. Using the breath as a guide, the entire body is scanned. When an area of tension is noticed, the mind sends the breath to that area, illuminating the sensation, and moving on to the next. The practice continues until the body becomes fully relaxed and the breath returns to neutral (Kabat-Zinn, 1990, p. 12).

Yoga movement starts with Pranayama or Breath Control. Gates (2015) used techniques that energized the body, stimulated the brain and calmed the mind, explaining, "In these practices we use the breath in specific ways for different effects – particularly for supporting sympathetic/parasympathetic balance and self-regulation" (p. 2) and she instructed:

> Begin in the here and now, noticing the breath and never forcing it. Increase the length of breath gradually. If anything feels inappropriate, do not do it! Observe what is happening in the body. First notice areas of openness and ease, than areas of tension and holding. Then feel into the quality of the breath – the rhythm, texture, feeling of the breath as it flows in and out of the body. Do you feel energized or calm, or jumpy? Now observe the thinking mind. What is present? Fixated? Spacious? Just notice without analyzing or judging. Finally observe an emotional tone. Notice the quality and the narrative. Then bring the attention back to the body. This gives the opportunity to recognize what may be most beneficial in terms of bringing balance. (p. 2-3)

Having connected with full body awareness, attention turns to the feeling tones, beginning with Pranayamas (breath control). Energy, calm, balance and focus were the Pranayamas to choose from. *Energizing practices* focused on inhalation, done in stages, combined with broad movements in a standing asana. *Calming practices* emphasized exhalations in stages combined with forward bending and twisting asanas. *Balancing practice* focused on stabilizing the breath with equal length inhalation and exhalation with combined with a neutral asana (sitting or lying down). *Focusing practice* cultivated relaxation and alertness by imagining the breath as it flowed through the body, in a lying down or standing asana doing bilateral movements (opposite arm to leg). Refer to Appendix D for full descriptions and instructions of the pranayamas and asanas. (Gates, 2015, p. 3-4).

Focus then turns to the body. Connection to the body begins with gentle movements. Kabat-Zinn (1996) explained that yoga was "never about accomplishment or perfection or even about technique itself. Nor was it about turning one's body into an elaborate pretzel" (p. 88). In his work with chronic pain sufferers, he discovered his clients' fear of yoga and he encouraged them to "start wherever they find themselves, with an attitude of gentleness and kindness toward themselves" (p.88).

According to Cushman (2014), "When you're practicing mindful yoga, your emphasis is not on *what* you're doing but on *how* you're doing it. You're practicing in a way that is intimately in touch with your body, your breath, your heart, and your mind" (p. xvi). The importance of practicing Mindful yoga for those in recovery is that it teaches an individual to become intimately aware of his or her body. Mind-altering substances have been found to negatively affect the body and mind. Yoga could provide a way to heal the body from such ailments as headaches and respiratory problems that may have hindered exercise (Pietrangello, 2014, www.healthline.com, n/p). Yoga could provide a way to heal the mind, reversing anhedonia and restoring a desire to exercise (Surguladze, 2003, p. 55).

Yin yoga is a gentle form of yoga. It is the art of holding a pose at least 3 minutes and as long as 5. The breath is controlled while holding the pose. The hold allows for gentle, thorough stretching of an area of the body while the stillness provides space for meditation during the pose. Feeling tones are to be noticed. Thoughts and memories are identified and redirected. As space opens up in the body, it also opens up in the mind. As described by Cushman (2014), "Another useful tool for awakening to sensations is to settle into a chosen pose for an extended period of time so that deeper and deeper layers of your body and psyche can begin to reveal themselves...On a physical level, a yin yoga practice allows the deeper layers of the body—the denser, tighter tissues of ligaments and connective tissue—to release in a way that they don't have time to do when we are moving more quickly" (p. 56-57).

## Feelings

Yoga is useful in locating any pleasant, unpleasant and neutral feeling tones in the body while also revealing the pleasant, unpleasant, and neutral feeling tones attached to the thoughts, and memories flowing through the mind. As reported by Hanson, et al., (2009), "Stimuli that evoke a pleasant or unpleasant feeling tone stir up more brain activity than neutral tones do, because there is more to think about and to respond to" (p. 115). Gates (2015) introduced meditative techniques that regulate the feeling tones during yoga. Known as Resourcing, it could be used to cultivate self-regulation by evoking positive states of well-being. The techniques could be used as way to train the mind to find the "direct sensory/somatic experience without storyline or interpretation" and described as follows:

- Orienting – orienting yourself to where you are in space, location geographically and bodily, knowing where you are who you are with and where the exits are, etc., so you feel more comfortable and at ease.

- Grounding – feeling where your body comes into contact with the earth, your feet, the seat, pacing hands on belly center, breathing into belly.

- Calling in your teachers, mentors and guides – inviting them into the space with you as you practice. Drawing on those streams of energy as a source of support.

- Internal resource – sensations, a place in body that feel neutral or comforting, a special place to go to in your imagination, feelings of empowerment, compassion.

- External resource – relying on a friend or loved one reaching out in a moment of need. (p. 1-2)

The resources provided a sense of stability and provided a way to navigate unpleasant experiences with more ease and comfort.

**Mind**

"A body badly burned by alcohol does not often recover overnight nor do twisted thinking and depression vanish in a twinkling" (Alcoholics Anonymous, 1955, p.133). Yin Yoga provides release of tension in the body. "But it's also a meditation in itself, in which your arising experience percolates through the filter of your sustained attention. As the deep tissues of the body let go, they release memories, emotions and dreams" (Cushman, 2014, p. 57). Recalling that *process* identifies a thought, and *content* identifies meaning attached to the thought (Levine, 2007, p. 135-136), the body is now providing deeper levels of process and content investigation. Moving that awareness from the external (body) to the internal (process and content) is known as interiorization, and Hartranet (2003) explained, "As interiorization proceeds, consciousness withdraws the senses from gross external objects, turning instead to subtle internal ones. Perfect discipline directed at the perceptual process itself means interiorizing to the point at which the subtle aspects of sensing become visible in consciousness" (p. 57). The discipline he spoke of was that of consistency in the practices of Mindful meditation and yoga.

## Mental Qualities

Siegel (1999) explained that, "Emotion is fundamentally linked to the same circuitry that is responsible for creating meaning and value for mental representations. It is no surprise that particular emotions become associated with particular states of mind" (p. 226). Mental qualities are developed from lived experiences. The metal qualities of anger, fear, depression, and anxiety have been identified as common qualities of newly sober individuals, cultivated during the years of substance abuse. The founders of Alcoholics Anonymous, 1952, elucidated, "The alcoholic is like a tornado roaring in his way through the lives of others. Hearts are broken. Sweet relationships are dead. Affections have been uprooted" (p 82.).

The road to recovery includes cultivation of positive emotions. Siegel (1999) reported that, "Emotional 'dysregulation' can be seen as impairments in this capacity to allow flexible and organized responses that are adaptive to the internal and external environment" (p. 241). Emotional "dysregulation" could be reversed through Mindfulness practices. Resourcing (Gates, 2015, p. 2), Yin yoga (Cushman, 2014, p. 57) and Mindful meditation (Levine, 2007, p. 135) provide the ability to regulate emotions resulting in more flexible and organized responses to the environment.

### Effects on Sex Life

Addicts and alcoholics often equated sex with love (Braun-Harvey, 2009, p. 52). Many substance abusers have never experienced sober sex. In addition, a true connection with another human being was difficult with the brain being impaired by substances. While leading a group in recovery, Braun-Harvey (2009) elaborated:

> Many of you have probably been in situations where you were using alcohol and/or drugs as part of your sexual behavior. You may have used drugs to try something new sexually. You may have gotten drunk or high to just feel sexual or to do something that you might be too embarrassed or anxious to do sober. You may have gotten high to feel more connected with your partner. You may have gotten high in order to tolerate or forget a terrible sexual experience. You probably had many different circumstances for being high before, during, or after sex. (p. 52)

Once sober, it becomes important for the individual to understand sex, sexuality, lust and love. It is also important to learn how to have healthy and enjoyable sex in sobriety. Braun-Harvey (2009) continued, "It takes a serious commitment to maintain your sobriety and recovery combined with addressing the emotions connected with attractions, desire, sexuality, and love" (p. 53).

Levine (2007) believed that "sexuality is not inherently anything other than a natural biological human experience that is totally neutral" (p. 85). However it did evoke pleasure on a sensory level and an emotional level. He continued, "The issue here is not sexual energy itself, then, since that is an innately human characteristic. The difficulty we face lies in our inner relationship of attachment to pleasure" (p. 85).

Awareness of the attachment one had to pleasure is the key to enjoyable sober sex. Attractions, desires, crushes, and lustful thoughts are emotionally charged mental qualities. The Mindfulness practices have given a sober person tools to address the emotionally charged mental qualities while cultivating a new inner relationship of their attachment to pleasure.

Application of Yin yoga provides two important elements to recovery. The first element is reparation to the body. Many people in recovery have been sedentary for many years. Bodily functions fluctuate during use and abstinence. Internal organs hold onto toxins that may cause illness and pain. Emotions fluctuate wildly. Sobriety brings vulnerability to an individual, manifesting in low self-esteem, unhealthy body image and fear. Physical challenges present themselves with sobriety, such a labored breathing and headaches (Kuhn, et al., 2008, p. 272-273). Nurturing the body back to health is a very important component of recovery. Yoga provides room to "befriend your body" (Cushman, 2014, p. 153). Yoga strengthens and tones muscles, oxygenates the blood, and activates the ANS, which elevates mood. Cushman (2014) explained, "In your yoga practice you can nurture your ability to be with your physical challenges—that funky hip, that vulnerable neck—not as problems but as parts of you that particularly need care. (p. 157). Metta could be applied to the body. Through the gate of yoga asana, Cushman went on to describe how to "attune your body to create an inner environment that's supportive of metta meditation and how to carry it out into your life and relationships" (p. 154). Just as phrases of loving-kindness had been directed towards self and others in meditation, metta messages of friendliness were to be directed towards parts of the body that needed care: *"May you feel at ease, aching hip, May you be at peace clenched jaw"* (p. 160).

The second important element of Yin yoga is the regulation of emotions. Pranayama with Resourcing (Gates, 2015, p.1-2) and Yin yoga (Cushman, 2013, p. 56-57) regulate emotions by paying attention to sensations in the body and to reactions to those sensations as they pass through the mind. According to Cushman (2014), there are exercises that focus on the pelvic floor which help regulate emotions attached to that sensitive area of the body. The exercises illuminate and enhance sensations that could lead to better sex. Calling it *Pulsing the Perineum*, she described its purpose in this way:

> Channel your attention to the pelvic floor—in particular the perineum, the triangle of muscle located just between the anus and the genitals...The root chakra, in yogic psychology, is often linked to feelings of security, groundedness and safety. And whether or not you believe this correlation between the energy body and the psyche, you may find that moving your attention into this part of the body—connecting intimately with the felt sense of it subtle pulsation—is a powerful way to draw your attention away from the scampering gerbils in your head. (p. 215)

While in a sitting or lying down asana, attention is directed to that area. Closing the eyes, the mind could sense the pelvic floor releasing, allowing the mind to rest in the perineum. She suggested "living inside the pulsation of the perineum" and intensifying its action by adding movement—a slight lifting and toning of the pelvic floor and the perineum. "Often taught forcefully as a contraction of the anus or vaginal muscles, it can be felt more subtly—and ultimately more powerfully—as a delicate lift as if tugging upward on the center of a spider web" (p. 216). By adding the intention of joy and rapture to the pulsing of the perineum, sensations of the genital area could be enhanced emotionally and physically. The dedication to Mindful practices enables an individual to call forth positive emotions when needed (Hanson et al., 2009, p.198). Sex could then be experienced with attention to the breath and body in present-time awareness, and with positive intention that focused on the genitals for a more enjoyable experience.

71

## Conclusions about Mindfulness Practices

Meditation is an important foundation of Mindfulness practices (Levine, 2009, p. 39). The formal training for meditation trains individuals to direct attention and awareness to the breath, the body, feeling tones, and mind states that arise. Diligent practice allows for Mindfulness to be present throughout the day. Having the intention of loving-kindness provides pleasurable feelings to a newly sober mind by releasing DA into the pleasure center of the brain. Continued meditation practices have been shown to increase gray matter in the hippocampal area of the brain, located in the pleasure center of the brain to regulate emotions (Holzel, et al., 2011, p. 36). Consistent meditation practices are needed to effect permanent change to the brain and thought processes because physiological changes in the brain are minimal unless practiced for at least two months on a daily basis (Holzel, et al., 2011 p. 36).

Yoga practices aid in improving the body/mind connection through breath regulation while providing energy through body movement (Gates, 2015, p.1-2). Addicts and alcoholics have often been sedentary for years and yoga provides a way to introduce body movement and body awareness to a sober individual for successful recovery. Yin yoga provides a gentle way to practice yoga without injury and it provides deep muscle and tissue healing while uncovering deep emotions and memories in the mind. Controlled breathing helps to regulate the SNS and PNS (Cushman, 2014, p.79-80). An intention of loving-kindness directed at specific parts of the body creates a new relationship with an ailing body. Yoga practices help to heal much of the physical damage brought about from substance abuse.

By combining Mindfulness practices with sex a more positive attitude could be brought into sober sexual experiences. With a toned body from yoga, and present-time awareness from meditation, positive energy could flow through the body and the mind. Invoking joy and rapture into the mind could manifest the mind-state of happiness. Pulsing the perineum could add new sensations to the genitals. Utilizing all the tools could bring enjoyment to sober sex. It was reasonable to assume that since Mindfulness practices helped regulate emotions and brought whole body awareness to sober individuals, the practices could be considered a viable solution for finding enjoyment during sex without using mind-altering substances.

## Chapter Summary

In summary, the chapter reviewed the effects of mind-altering substances to the body and the brain and their negative effects on the sex lives of substance abusers. The substances in the review were marijuana, stimulants, depressants and alcohol. The review included the history of the substances, and effects to the body, mind and spirit. Physiological and psychological aspects were explored. The chapter then reviewed the effects of Mindfulness practices on the body and the brain and their positive effects on the sex lives of people in recovery. The Mindfulness practices in review were meditation and Yin yoga. The literature provided the history of the practices, along with the effects to the body, mind and spirit. Physiological and psychological results were explored from scientific and spiritual perspectives.

The research suggested that sex in sobriety was frightening. Substance abuse caused emotional and physical difficulties. Mindful meditation practices helped train the mind to redirect difficult emotions into positive emotions, and strengthened the mind to focus on present-time awareness when needed. Mindful yoga healed the body, connecting it with the breath, activating the nervous system, and energizing the spirit.

The Centers for Disease Control, and the National Drug Counsel were among the sites reviewed for mind-altering substances. The Center For Mindfulness, The IASHS, AMA, Noah Levine, Dr. Daniel Siegel, Dr. Jon Kabat-Zinn and more supplied information about Mindfulness practices.

The following chapter will explore the relationship between sobriety and Mindfulness practices and the possibility that combining them could result in enjoyable sober sex.

# Chapter 3 - Methodology

## Introduction

The lived experience of people in recovery facing the difficulties of sober sex and finding solutions to those difficulties was the focus of the study. The research was aimed at the dissemination of specific narratives about sex: What sex was like while using mind-altering substances, what happened once the subject became sober with a focus on sex and finally describing the results of utilizing Mindfulness practices to change the sexual experiences in sobriety. A collaborative narrative combined the stories to be included in the findings.

## Rationale for Research Approach

A Qualitative Research Study was chosen using a Narrative Method to compile findings. The Labovian Structure was used for coding. Created by Labov and Waletsky (1967) it was described by Harper and Thompson (2012) in the following way:

> This involves seeking particular aspects of a story, including orientation, complicating action and evaluation. At most the simplified level, the orientation is the 'scene-setting' of a particular narrative (stating where or when a situation occurred). The complicating action is the essence of the story and the reason for it being told, and the evaluating is the point at which the story is concluded and summarized. (p. 168)

The *orientation* was the physical and psychological narrative about the subject's sex life during their using and in recovery. The *complicating action* was sobriety itself and the discovery of difficulties that occur during sober sex. *Evaluation* explored the need of the subject to find a solution to those difficulties.

It was important to record the lived experiences of sober individuals who had an understanding of the challenges of sober sex and who were also on a journey of healing, using Mindfulness practices that include meditation and yoga. It was also important to record the findings due to the lack of empirical research about sober sex. The subject of recovery is clouded in mystery since sobriety is generally an anonymous endeavor. Answers to questionnaires and narratives provided by people in recovery brought legitimacy to the subject of sober sex, bringing awareness to problems related to sober sex and offering a viable solution to experiencing enjoyable sober sex.

## Research Setting and Context

Since the study involved sexual encounters past and present, the studies were to be conducted in the participants' natural settings. Primary natural setting was the subject's home, although one participant chose varied locations, as described in a narrative. The context was to describe sober sex before and after the application of Mindfulness techniques. In order to maintain authenticity for the participants as they engaged in sexual activities, the natural setting was the choice of the subject.

## Research Sample and Data Sources

The research sample was made up of four adults, all in recovery, all practicing Mindful meditation and yoga. The sample was chosen by face-to-face inquiry and interviews from volunteers found in 12-step meetings. The focus of the study was to gather stories from four sober, adult individuals who had already been practicing Mindfulness as a means to enjoy sober sex. Along with the researcher, three sober adults who matched the criteria were chosen to participate: A 61-year old male with 21 years of sobriety and began practicing Mindful meditation and yoga within the last six months, a 55-year old female with 6 years of sobriety and Mindfulness practices of over 17 years and a 50-year old female with 3 years in recovery and 3 years with Mindfulness practices. Narrative research was chosen for its design to focus on specific lived experiences from a small sampling of a population to impart pertinent ideas to professionals and laypersons. As Clandinin and Connelly (2000) explained:

> Select one or more individuals who have stories or life experiences to tell, and spend considerable time with them gathering their stories through multiple types of information. Research participants may record their stories in a journal or diary, or the researcher might observe the individuals...Collect information about the context of these stories. Narrative researchers situate individual stories within participants' personal experiences (their jobs, their homes), their culture (racial or ethnic), and their historical contexts (time and place). Analyze the participants' stories,

and then "restory" them into a framework that makes sense...Collaborate with participants by actively involving them in the research. As researchers collect stories, they negotiate relationships, smooth transitions, and provide ways to be useful to the participants. (p. 57)

Participants signed consent forms (Appendix F) in accordance with the Institutional Review Board (IRB) before participating in the study. The names of the participants were changed in order to protect their anonymity. All information gathered and exchanged will remain confidential. All journal entries and written narratives will remain the property of the participants. Final approval will to be given by the participants prior to its inclusion in the final draft of the dissertation.

## Data Collection Methods

Questionnaires were distributed (Appendix A) to provide information about age, gender, past and current sexual partner(s), length of time in sobriety and length of time of practicing Mindfulness. Narratives were then written from their memories and current events, describing details about having sex during their using, once sober and after applying Mindfulness to sober sex. Interviews were done privately, at their homes.

## Data Analysis Method

Information was categorized manually, using the Labovian Structure as shown in Figure 1 for identifying events along with a narrative of the experiences.

| Narrative | ABSTRACT: begins by providing context of what the story is about (journey of sober sex) |
|---|---|
| Narrative | ORIENTATION: here it emerges the who, what, where, when, why (person in recovery) |
| Narrative | The COMPLICATING ACTION: is the revelation of the concealment of events (difficulties in sober sex) |
| Narrative | The participant's EVALUATION: gives the reason for the action taken (wants a solution) |
| Narrative | RESULT: the participant describes sexual experiences pre- and post- recovery (character of participants) |
| Narrative | CODA: the participant summarizes, and brings the context back to the start (sober sex and Mindfulness) |

*Figure 1:* Labovian Structure

## Issues of Trustworthiness

To enhance the study, instructional guidelines for breath Resourcing was distributed to each participant, along with copies of loving-kindness meditation phrases that focus on the body and evoke joy and rapture (Appendices D and E). Narratives were to then focus on the lived experience as it related to sex before and after recovery. Daily journal entries had been requested to add to the dependability of the study. The sample was given a start date and an end date for the study that allowed for one month to complete the questionnaires and journals.

## Limitations and Delimitations

Given that Narrative Studies relied on recollections of past lived-experiences, and descriptions of present sensations and emotions, limitations were based on lack of scientific findings from the sample itself. Information gathered was subjective and therefore limited to descriptions of felt-sense experiences of the participants. Final results were based on the combined experiences of sober sex and Mindfulness from a small sampling of a larger whole.

Delimitations occurred from the final sample's ages. Subjects were aged 50 to 61. All participants resided in Los Angeles, CA. No restrictions were placed on length of sobriety or Mindfulness practices. The only requirements were to be sober and practicing Mindfulness.

Neither the limitations nor delimitations affected the transferability of the findings to the sober community as a whole. Neither limitation nor delimitations affected the transferability of the findings to the professional community as a useful addition to Treatment Facility curriculum or Addiction and Recovery Counseling as well as the field of Sexology.

## Summary

A Qualitative Study was conducted using a Narrative method. The sample was a group of four sober adults from ages 50-61 who matched the requirements of active sobriety and active practice of Mindful meditation and yoga. The focus of the study was sober sex. Narratives supplied the descriptions of sex before sobriety, the difficulties associated with sober sex and the felt-sense recollection of bringing

Mindful techniques into sober sexual experiences. Data collection was done using the Labovian Structure, as shown in Figure 1.

Limitations have been attributed to the lack of scientific data collection from the sample. All data was subjective and dependent on the story as told by each subject. A combined narrative provided the end result as representation for the larger body of sober people as a whole. Delimitations included an age range from 50-61 with all participants residing in Los Angeles, CA. The requirements for participating were active sobriety and active Mindfulness practices prior to enrolment.

A collaborative narrative combined with personal experience and those in the sample made the results of this study viable and transferable to a larger community of sober people and to professionals in the recovery field as a way to address sex in sobriety in Treatment Centers.

# Chapter 4 - Results

The research focused on the impact Mindfulness Practices might have on sober sex. Four people in recovery described what sex was like while using mind-altering substances, what happened once they got sober with a focus on sex, and finally describing the results of utilizing Mindfulness practices to change their sexual experiences in sobriety. Unlike previous studies on the challenges of sober sex conducted by Braun-Harvey (2009) and previous studies conducted by Kabat-Zinn (1990) and Hanson & Medius (2009) about the benefits of Mindfulness meditation and yoga, this study focused on the lived experiences of people in recovery who have applied Mindfulness practices to their sober sexual experiences.

This Qualitative Narrative study used a small sample to describe any changes to their sex lives in sobriety after applying Mindfulness. The study was used as a means to expand awareness of the difficulties that were inherent to sober sex and to provide a viable solution to be used as a method to overcome those difficulties. In addition, future use of the study was considered to generate ideas for further exploration into this underrepresented area of research.

The results were compiled from answers to the questionnaire in Appendix A along with narratives from the participants. The Labovian Structure as shown in Appendix B was used to locate patterns and themes in the sample. The narratives from each participant were broken down into six categories. Appendix B represented the findings of the Labovian Structure Method with an Abstract explaining the sex lives from childhood through to sobriety, an Orientation describing the parameters of the participants, the Complicating Actions detailing the challenges of sober sex, an Evaluation of the challenges, a Result from complications to solution and a Coda revealing final analyses. A collaborative narrative in Appendix C completed the study. The results from the study were then combined and recorded in the answers to the three research questions outlined in Chapter 1 with a discussion following.

According to the American Psychological Association (2011), "Personal communications may be private letters, memos, some electronic communications (e.g. e-mail or messages from non-archived discussions groups or electronic bulletin boards) personal interviews, telephone conversations, and the like...Cite personal communications in text only" (p. 179). Therefore, cited dialogue has been referenced in-text with an Appendix letter of A, B or C along with a page number and anonymous interviews have been referenced as personal communications dated 2015 in parentheses.

## Research Questions

Research question #1: How do sober adults recall their sexual experiences while they were still using mind-altering substances?

Using information provided in the questionnaire from Appendix A (A), interviews, and narratives from Appendix C (C) and the Labovian Structure results from Appendix B (B), all four participants reported disruptions in their childhood experiences including divorce (#P3, B, p. 107 & #P4, B, p.108), sexual abuse (#P2, #P3, B, p. 105-

107), alcoholism (#P2, B, p. 105 #P4,, B. p.108), and death of a parent (#P4, B. p. 108).

None of the participants attributed their drug use to the disruptions at home, although one participant mentioned, "I had a lot of rage towards my mother. She sent me to boarding school because she couldn't handle me. That's where I smoked pot for the first time. It was just what the doctor ordered! I loved it. I felt so calm and peaceful for the first time in a long time" (#P1, B, p. 104). All four participants reported their first use of mind-altering substances during adolescence: one was age 14 (#P1 B, p. 104), two were age 13 (#P2, B, p. 105, #P3. B, p.107), and one was age 15 (#P4, B, p. 108). One participant (#P1, B, p. 104) had been prescribed a psychotropic medication at age 10. The psychotropic medication had been stopped prior to the participant's alcohol and marijuana use. Alcohol was the first substance used by two of the participants (#P2, B, p. 105, & #P4. B. p.108), and marijuana by two of the participants (#P1,B, p. 104 #P3, B. p. 107). 100% of the participant became poly-substance abusers with all four having used the following: marijuana, alcohol, cocaine, heroin, methamphetamine, Ecstasy, prescription opiates, and sleep aids.

All of the participants admitted to masturbating before they reached the age of 6. None of the participants attributed their sexual behaviors to the disruptions at home. The study revealed that 100% of the subjects used sex to get close to people. As P4 reported:

> I gave a hand job to my boyfriend and thought I was going to go to hell! He wanted more from me. I wanted him to love me. I was afraid if I didn't go all the way, he would leave me. I lost my virginity to him the next weekend. I figured right then, as long as I'm already going to hell, I might as well keep going! I never looked back. (C, p. 112)

As described by #P1, "Lost my virginity at age 15, fell in love at age 16. We were 'making love,' for indeed love went with every caress and act of intercourse" (C, p. 113) Two participants (#P2, #P3) reported using substances during their first sexual experiences with another person. One participant explained, "In junior high school I had my first homosexual encounter. It was with a schoolmate. We were high and we kissed and dry humped each other. I was so scared but it felt so good" (#P3, B, p. 107) and another stated, "I thought I was a better lover when I was intoxicated. I think there was some truth in me feeling 'less inhibited' when I was drinking, especially when initiating sex" (#P2, B, p. 106).

According to 100 % of the participants, the progression of drug and alcohol use led to progression in sexual activity. Each participant described humiliating events, and dangerous behaviors while under the influence. As detailed by #P1:

> I was teaching at an art school and the drugs and alcohol and sex escalated. I had many one-night stands thinking my prowess in bed would make them love me. My goal was to give excellent blowjobs because men were more interested in me that way. Got married and drugs and alcohol were

more important. Sex was awful. Divorced, age 32, got into the BDSM world. Gave myself to over 20 Doms, many angry men. As I got more savvy, I became a true submissive, humiliated and tortured. Loved being made to do their wishes-NO ORGASMS. My drinking and coke use made me delusional in terms of my sexual prowess and I allowed myself to get into many dangerous situations all over the world, being a slave, blood and knife play, fisting, housed in a cage. Many offered money and I took it. (B, p. 104)

As described by #P2:

I remember feeling "bolder" and somehow more fun as a sex partner. But I also remember times when I'd pass out in the middle of making love, or feel numb either emotionally or physically, making climaxing difficult or impossible. Which lead to faking an orgasm at times, but for who? And to what end? This just caused a feeling of not being authentic, which I loathe. So the thought of being a better lover or more fun, however fleeting or untrue, really lead me into a downward spiral of feeling bad about myself from passing out, feeling numb or inauthentic. Which of course lead to more drinking and distancing myself from feeling bad about myself. What a vicious cycle. (B. p. 110)

#P3 stated:

I lived in a commune in Marin County. I sold pot for a living. My drinking escalated and so did my sex life. We had parties and orgies and I got really good at blowjobs. That is still my favorite thing, actually.

So much of that time is a blur. It got weird with HIV and AIDS so blackouts were really scary. I remember waking up with guys I didn't remember meeting and panicking for weeks while I got tested. It was a crazy time. San Francisco was a drag so I moved to Los Angeles. I was such a whore! Got busted in Griffith Park giving a guy a blowjob! The fucking cop watched the whole thing, probably got off! I was a registered sex offender until last year! My drugging got so bad...finally, I couldn't get it up and I didn't even want to. (B, p. 108)

As #P4 described:

I worked at a bank by day, and drank, drugged and punk rock and rolled at night. I moved in with a drug dealer. Bruises, broken noses, cops and robberies were all a part of that relationship! Next, a Junky, musician who never held a job and helped me cop a heroin habit! We imploded and I slept around and partied until I found my Porn Star! We smoked crack and drank and fought and laughed and he gave me STDs and he left. I kept drinking and sleeping around. I remember trying to count how many people I slept with. I got to 25 and stopped counting. I felt so guilty and dirty. I found love again in Paris. A train wreck! Drinking took away my ability to orgasm and there was lots of violence and he left me to drink alone. So I did! I began having heart pains and the shakes. I threw up every day and pissed on myself every night (B, p. 109)

All four participants reported being less inhibited while intoxicated. Two of the participants (#P1, #P2, personal communication, 2015) reported that drinking and drugs made them feel as though they were better lovers while intoxicated. Two of the participants reported developing physical ailments due to drug and alcohol abuse, (P2, heart attack, and P4, tremors), two reported legal issues (#P3, sexual offender, and #P4, drunk in public, personal communication, 2015), three reported feelings of guilt or humiliation (#P1, #P2, #P4, personal communication, 2015) while three of the participants reported they did not have orgasms due to drug and alcohol abuse (#P1, #P2, #P4, personal communication, 2015). 100% reported having multiple sex partners, with 75% of the participants having engaged in sex with complete strangers. Only one participant reported Domestic Violence (#P4), stating, "I was never one to sit around and get hit. I fought back and paid for it, the worst being a broken nose" (B, p. 109). Finally, all four subjects stated their reasons for having sex was to feel loved and to show love to another person.

Considering the emergent patterns and themes found in the sample's narratives, additional research is needed. In the recovery field, further investigation into the reasons for addiction would be needed considering 100% of the participants reported that family disruptions were not to blame for their alcohol and drug use. Further research is needed in the sexology field due to the emergent theme that addicts and alcoholics use sex to give and receive love, a belief reported to be true for all four participants.

Research question #2: How did getting sober change your sexual experiences?

When asked, all four subjects reported fear during sober sex, with #P2 stating, "I remember being so scared of so many things when I first got sober. Everything seemed so new and different." #P4 revealed, "I met a guy in my first week of sobriety. We had sex on our first 'date,' my M. O. I was submissive and fearful because I did not know how to behave" (B, p. 104).

Two subjects reported lack of pleasure while having sober sex, with #P1 stating, "My first sober sex experience was with [my old Master]. The sex was horrible, it hurt and I was never aroused. BDSM was worse. I could not tolerate it. I had straight sex with a friend and it was the worst experience I have ever had" (B., p. 104) while #P3 reported, "Sex with my partner was dull" (B, p. 108). Intimacy with another person was difficult for 100 % of the participants. #P1 reported that after having such bad experiences, "I did not have sex for 4 years in sobriety. It was a lonely time" (B, p. 104). As described by #P4, "Talking about our sexual experiences was not something that [my partner] and I were used to, so bringing up my fears about how to be an intimate partner, without alcohol, was not something I was comfortable doing with [my partner]" (B, p. 109) #P3 stated, "I lack intimacy with [my partner] and outside relationships only satisfy my sexual urges, not my relationship concerns" (B, p. 108). According to #P2, "Sex did not bring intimacy. Sex was embarrassing and scary. I created messy relationships in sobriety because I relied on sex to feel love and it backfired every time" (B, p. 106).

Results of this study suggested the emotional and mental difficulties in sexual experiences in the early stages of sobriety. None of the participants revealed information regarding physical difficulties that might have occurred from their drug and alcohol abuse. Further research is needed to address any physical limitations that result from drug and alcohol abuse in order to rule out medical conditions independent of addiction, or to locate concomitant symptoms that effect sexual experiences.

Research Question #3: What details can sober adults provide regarding changes in their sex lives after applying Mindfulness practices?

The questionnaires as seen in Appendix A (personal communication, 2015) revealed that 3 participants (#P1, #P3, #P4) practiced a form of Mindful mediation and yoga after entering recovery, while one participant (#P2) had been practicing Mindful meditation and yoga prior to getting sober. One hundred percent of the participants reflected changes in their sober sexual experiences after applying Mindfulness techniques learned from the practices.

#P1 admitted:

> I have never used the term "mindfulness" as it related to sex. Spontaneity and the excitement of impending sex have always been paramount. But when I am practicing my AA principals, meditating and living in the moment, and having a fit and attractive body, I feel very sexy. I guess you can call it "mindfulness." I do know that after I met [my partner] I had the best sex of my life! I was able to

tell him everything I wanted and was turned on by hearing him tell me likewise. (personal communication, 2015)

#P3 explained that meditation had always helped to suppress his anger but, "It never occurred to me to use it with sex until it was suggested for this study (personal communication, 2015). #P3 then explained that after applying loving-kindness mantras to meditation practice and integrating the rapture and joy mantras for two weeks, "I am actually feeling closer to [my partner] than I have in a long time. It is helping me want to have sex with him. And the rapture and joy mantras have really elevated the excitement a bit for me" (personal communication, 2015). According to #P4:

I needed to learn that sleeping with someone did not mean love. I never knew how to have a satisfying and intimate relationship with someone without sleeping with him. Once I connected with someone on a non-sexual but intimate level, I chose to have sober sex. It was sensual, and gentle and I was completely aware the entire time. We were cuddling and kissing and I can have orgasms...I still have bouts of fear surrounding sex. Mindfulness practices help me tap into those fears at any given moment. I can then see the truth of the fear, the feeling, whatever. The rest takes care of itself. I never feel angry or guilty during or after sex anymore. It is wonderful! (personal communication, 2015)

#P2, having practiced Mindfulness meditation and yoga for 13 years before entering recovery asserted:

> What was scary is that I wasn't sure how to "be" as a lover. One of my fears was learning how to be an intimate, sexual being. I associated the thoughts of being "fun," "uninhibited" and "a better lover" with alcohol. So I feared that I would not or could not be these things as a sober lover. Of course the truth was I was not necessarily any of these things, these were just thought patterns associated with drinking and sex. Mindfulness was helping me stay sober...It was also invaluable to helping me walk through the "new" experience of making love, sober. My practice helped me slow my thoughts down, reinhabit my body so I could be as fully present and in the moment as possible when making love...This translated into me being able to notice physical sensations and pleasure during sex, that many times had been lost when I was inebriated. (personal communication, 2015)

All four participants reported that changes in their sober sexual experiences were positive in nature when the Mindfulness practices were utilized. One hundred percent reported improvement in intimacy with a partner. Fifty percent of the participants (#P2, #P4, personal communication, 2015) applied techniques before and during sober sex, while the other 50% (#P1, #P3, personal communication, 2015) reported using Mindfulness before but not during sober sex. The descriptions of combining sober sex with Mindfulness were as follows: "The most enjoyable sex I ever had" (#P1, B, p.104), "Our love making intensified" (#P2, B, p. 107), "Our closeness is growing and I am enjoying it much more" (#P3, B, p. 108), and "Now I have sober sex by choice, with awareness and enjoyment" (#P4, B, p. 110).

The results of the study suggested that Mindfulness meditation and yoga create positive changes to sober sex practices for individuals in recovery while creating a better connection with a sexual partner when applying present-time awareness, breath awareness and felt-sense awareness during sober sex. Further studies are needed in the field of recovery to explore greater populations of sober people to include other cultures, other races, the prison populations, and members of families with strong religious values. The field of sexology would benefit from further research to a broader range of sober sex practices including sex workers and those in poly-amorous relationships.

## Patterns and Themes

The patterns and themes produced from this study revealed similarities among all four participants regarding sex before and after sobriety. Many addicts and alcoholics believe that sex and love are interchangeable (Braun-Harvey, 2009). As Table 1 demonstrates, 100% of the participants held the belief that sex equaled love. In addition, all four participants reported a form of self-imposed celibacy due to excessive drug and alcohol use. According to #P1, "Humiliated and delusional about sexual prowess, I gave up sex altogether and drank and drugged 24/7." #P2 reported, "Marriage was strained, with no sex, no orgasms, and a straying mind." #P3 stated "My drinking and drugging got so bad...I couldn't get it up and I didn't even want to. I was done" and #P4 admitting, "No orgasms. No sex. Just drinking."

Additional patterns and themes emerged among the participant after getting sober. The study revealed changes to sober sex practices for 100% of the participants (Table 1). Seventy-five percent of the participants engaged in sex without the need to give or receive love, (#P1, #P2, #P3) and 75% of the participants engaged in sex to demonstrate love (#P1, #P2, #P4). The study revealed emotional changes for 100% of the participants. Results showed that all four participants no longer held the belief that sex and love were interchangeable and reported they could feel love without having to demonstrate it by engaging in sex.

Table 1
*The Meaning of Sex and Love*

| | |
|---|---|
| *SEX = LOVE*F #P1, #P2, #P3, #P4 | 100% used sex to demonstrate love |
| *SEX & DRUGS = LOVE*F #P1, #P2, #P3 | 75% used drugs to have sex to demonstrate love |
| *SEX = SEX* D #P1, #P2, #P3, #P4 F #P1, #P3 | 100% engaged in sex to demonstrate sex 50% engaged in sex to demonstrate |
| *SEX & DRUGS = ACCEPTANCE*F #P3 | 25% used drugs and sex for acceptance |
| *LOVE = SEX*D #P1, #P2, #P4 | 75% felt love and chose to engage in sex |
| *DRUGS = SEX & NO LOVE*F #P1, #P2, #P3 | 75% had sex without feeling love |
| *DRUGS = NO SEX & NO LOVE*F #P1, #P2, #P3, #P4 | 100% stopped having sex and feeling love |
| *LOVE = LOVE*D #P1, #P2, #P3, #P4 | 100% felt love without demonstrating it with sex |

The subjects are represented with codes #P1, #P2, #P3, #P4.
F - This symbol represents beliefs before sobriety
D - This symbol represents beliefs after Sobriety
Many addicts and alcoholics believe that sex and love are interchangeable.
Recovery helps to cultivate new beliefs about sex and love.

Table 2 demonstrates patterns and themes for sex in sobriety before and after the utilization of Mindfulness practices. The study revealed that, before applying Mindfulness techniques, all four participant experienced emotional challenges during sober sex, which included fear and lack of intimacy as well as physical challenges that included painful sex (#P1) and an inability to have orgasms (#P1, #P2, #P4). The study suggested that 100% of the participants experienced positive changes to their sober sex experiences after applying the Mindfulness techniques.

Table 2

*The Impact of Mindfulness Practices on Sober Sexual Experiences*

| | | |
|---|---|---|
| P1 | D Painful. D Humiliating. D No orgasms D "Scary" | W Feel joy by giving body as Masochist to Sadist. W Orgasms come quickly and feel better. W "Most enjoyable sex I have ever had." |
| P2 | D Frightening D Intimidating D No orgasms D "Don't know how to be an intimate, sexual being" | W The discovery that "I am enough." W "Notice physical sensations and pleasure during sex." W "Mindfulness has given me confidence during sex" |
| P3 | D Increased sex drive. D No intimacy. D Sex with partner dull. D "Afraid of being unfulfilled" | W Elevated excitement with partner. W Acceptance of partner's "vanilla sex life." W Feel closer to partner, increasing desire for sex with him. |
| P4 | D Slept around for affection. D "Hated" having sex. D No orgasms. D Scared and intimidated | W Stopped sleeping around. W Connected with a person on an intimate level. W Remained aware during sex. W Began to enjoy having sex. |

The subjects are represented as codes #P1, #P2, #P3, #P4

D - This symbol represents sober sex Pre-Mindfulness

W - This symbol represents sober sex Post-Mindfulness

Sexual experiences become a challenge for an individual in recovery.

Mindfulness practices have been shown to effect changes to sober sexual experiences.

## Patterns

In this study a pattern is "a combination of qualities, acts, tendencies, etc., forming a consistent or characteristic arrangement" (dictionary.refernce.com, n.d., n/p).

The belief that sex and love were interchangeable was the discernible pattern for all four participants before recovery (C, p. 112). Braun-Harvey (2009) described it as, "Using drugs and alcohol to express love to a partner or to a receive expressions of love from a partner. (For example, wanting to feel close, wanting to feel loved, needing to be touched, wanting to feel comforted, wanting to express my love to my partner)" (p. 53-54). Two of the participants reported feeling "...bolder and somehow more fun as a sex partner" (#P2, B, p. 107), "...thinking that my prowess in bed would make me a better lover" (#P1, B, p. 104) while the other two reported, "...I got drunk and slept with guys at parties. I just wanted to be loved" (#P4, B, p. 109), and "...a gay boy with a steady girlfriend, having drunk sex showed my love for her" (#P3, B, p.108).

Another pattern that emerged came after the participants became sober. One hundred percent of the participants reported intimacy difficulties with a partner, with #P1 reporting:

> As an active alcoholic my greatest sexual and romantic joy came from serving my Master and taking all his administered torture and humiliation. Now that I am sober, I do not care for humiliation; the sex and abusive sex felt awful. (B, p. 104)

#P2 stated, "One of my fears was learning how to be an intimate, sexual being" (B, p. 106), while #P3 reported, "I go outside of the relationship often. I still want intimacy with [my partner]" (B, p. 108). #P4 asserted, "And I never knew how to have a satisfying and intimate relationship with someone without sleeping with him" (B, p. 108).

Patterns related to utilizing Mindfulness practices during sober sex resulted in positive changes for all four participants. Results from the Labovian Structure (Appendix B) showed changes in the meanings of sex and love for 100% of the participants, and all four participants reported improvements in intimacy with their partners.

## Themes

For this study a theme is defined as "a subject of discourse, discussion, meditation, or composition; topic" (dictionary.reference.com, n. d., n/p). Regarding sex for newly sober individuals, the theme of fear was revealed. #P4 referred to sober sex as "embarrassing and frightening" (personal communication, 2015). #P2 stated, "Having sober sex was frightening and intimidating at times, because I didn't know how it would be, how I would be" (personal communication, 2015). As #P1 reported, "I was 48 years old, lost in a strange world without drugs or alcohol. It was scary" (personal communication, 2015). #P3 described having a stronger sex drive in recovery that raised fears about never finding enjoyment in sober sex, reporting that, "It's not fulfilling. [My partner] has a low sex drive and is dull in bed. Outside relationships only satisfy my sexual needs, not my relationship needs" (personal communication, 2015).

Finding ways to improve sober sex was the underlying theme and the purpose of this study. The utilization of Mindfulness was shown to bring positive changes to sober sexual experiences for all four participants. After practicing Mindfulness and applying the techniques to sober sexual experiences, 50% of the participants referred to sober sex as being "enjoyable"' (#P1, B, p. 104 & #P4, B, p. 110). One participant described the improvement as "...gaining a comfort level with it...a confidence that came with letting the moments unfold during sober sex" (#P2, B, p. 107) and one participant explained, "The joy and rapture mantras have elevated the excitement a bit for me" (#P3, B. p. 107).

## Conclusion

The purpose of a narrative method of research was to study the lived-experience from a specific event asking one or more individuals to provide stories about their lives (Creswell, 2014, p. 13). "This information is then often retold or restoried by the researcher into a narrative chronology" (Creswell, 2014, p. 245). Three of the participants in this study were known to the researcher through Recovery meetings and volunteered to provide detailed narratives about sex before and after sobriety and their experiences of using Mindfulness practices for enjoyable sober sex. The researcher completed the sample, bringing the number of participants to four.

When qualitative research was done via narratives, Tannen & Alatis (2003) explained, "In the great majority of cases, the only information available on the nature of reported events is in the narrative itself" (p. 63). Since the study was conducted in a natural setting without the researcher present and results were subjective, the researcher used a Labovian Structure to assimilate information from questionnaires, narratives and interviews to compile more accurate results. As Hansen (2006) explained:

> The qualitative researcher has an obligation to be methodical in reporting sufficient details of data collection and the processes of analysis to permit others to judge the quality of the resulting product. Even when the report takes the form of a narrative, researchers must be sure that their "telling of the story" gives readers an accurate and complete picture of the research. (p. 58)

The narratives provided voices to an aspect of life, from a specific community, that has been underrepresented in the fields of Recovery and Sexology. The participants willingly told their stories in hopes of raising awareness of the difficulties of engaging in sober sex and the need to find solutions to enjoy sober sex.

The discovery of patterns and themes in this small sample of individuals in recovery were important in defining common difficulties to sober sex for a larger population as well as identifying a possible common solution to overcoming sober sex difficulties.

Before getting sober, it was revealed that of 100% of the participants held the belief that sex and love were interchangeable, with individuals engaging in sex to demonstrate love while they were using. After sobriety the overriding theme for 100% of the participants was fear of having sex without mind-altering substances. The underlying theme was that sex in sobriety was not pleasant and a strong desire for a solution was present.

The study revealed that all four participants had been practicing Mindfulness meditation and yoga to varying degrees. 100% of the participants reported improvement to their sober sex lives when Mindfulness techniques were applied.

# Chapter 5 - Conclusions and Recommendations

Braun-Harvey (2009) noted that although great strides have been made in treating men women who suffer from addiction, he found that sexuality is "marginalized and even made invisible. When sexuality is not directly and positively addressed in drug and alcohol treatment, it can contribute to treatment failure, relapse, and untold costs in the lives of addicts and their families" (p.3). While there has been limited literature covering the subject of sober sex (Kettleback, 1993), and a great deal of literature covering Mindful meditation and yoga (Kabat-Zinn, 1990, 1996, 2003), there is a lack of information identifying Mindfulness as a solution to overcoming difficulties associated with sober sex. A narrative study was used to capture the essence of the lived-experience of four individuals in recovery searching for a solution for change to enjoy sex in sobriety.

## Limitations

Due to the small sample size of three women and one man over the age of 50 residing in Los Angeles, CA, generalizations about all men or all women who are in recovery and practicing Mindfulness could not be conclusively drawn. The Labovian Structure method of research, which concluded with a collaborative narrative, helped limit bias in the interpretation of outcomes.

A larger sample size could have provided more accurate and generalized results. Due to the anonymous nature of people in recovery, many inquiries to prospective participants went unanswered. The ability to interview those in recovery who were under the age of 50 could have created a broader understanding of difficulties that arise during sober sex for young adults. Additionally, a larger sample of those who identify as LGBT, people with severe physical challenges, a sample with Alternative Sex lifestyles such as BDSM and fetishes and a sample that included heterosexual men could shed much needed light on alternate beliefs about sex and love along with a broader range of sober sex concerns.

## Areas for Future Research

It would be recommended that research continue on the subject of sex in sobriety. Living in recovery is more than abstaining from mind-altering substances. Living in recovery requires the individual to cultivate new ways to feel pleasure. Mind-altering substances create emotional attachments and patterns of sexual behaviors that are difficult to change once a person gets sober. Treatment Professionals could benefit from education in Mindfulness and its usefulness in affecting changes in emotional attachments and sexual behaviors. Mindfulness practices could then be considered as a viable, holistic solution to finding pleasure and enjoying sex without mind-altering substances.

Multi-cultural research would be recommended in order to explore emerging patterns and themes or lack, thereof on a larger scale.

A long-term study could determine the efficacy of combining Mindfulness practices with sober sex practices. Long-term studies could ascertain lasting benefits not only to sexual experiences, but overall well-being of an individual in recovery.

# REFERENCES

alcohol. (n.d.). Roget's 21st Century Thesaurus, Third Edition. Retrieved August 04, 2015, from Thesaurus.com website: http://www.thesaurus.com/browse/booze

Alcoholics Anonymous, (1952). Twelve steps and twelve traditions. New York NY: Alcoholics Anonymous World Services, Inc.

American Psychological Association. (Sixth Printing, 2011). Publication manual of the American psychological association. Washington, DC: American Psychological Association.

Anderson, P. B., Spruille, B., & Strano, D. A. (2005). The relationship between heavy episodic drinking, sexual assaulting and being sexually assaulted for southern urban university students. Electronic Journal Of Human Sexuality, 8(4). Retrieved from www.ejhs.org

Bauer, B., Kavrakovski, Z. Kostik, V. (2015). Marijuana once and today. II Congress of Pharmacists of Montenegro with International participation, 28-31 May 2015. Retrieved from http://eprints.ugd.edu.mk/ 13334/

Benzodiazepines – definition of benzodiazepines (December 2014) abouthealth.com. Retrieved from http://ptsd.about.com/od/glossary/g/Benzo.htm?utm_term =what%20is%20benzodiazepine&utmcontent=p1-main-2-title&utm_medium=sem&utm_source=msn&utm_campaign =adid-af1f04e7-5e13-4982-8209-a92ac6c5fc15-0 ab_mse_ocode-22846&ad=semD&an=msn_s&am=exact&q=what%20is%20 benzodiazepine&dqi=&o=22846&l=sem&qsrc=999&askid=a f1f04e7-5e13-4982-8209-a92ac6c5fc15-0-ab_mse9

Bhikkhu, T. (2008). Satipatthana sutta: The Foundations of Mindfulness/The Discourse on the Arousing of Mindfulness/Frames of Reference. Handful of Leaves (1) MN10. Retrieved from http://www.accesstoinsight.org/tipitaka/mn/index.html#mn.01 0.than

Biddulph, D., & Flynn, D. (2009). Teachings of the Buddha: The wisdom of the Dharma, from the Pali canon to the sutras. San Francisco, CA: Duncan Baird.

Bixler, J. (2011, October 19). More than 1 in 10 in U.S. take antidepressants. Retrieved March 30, 2015, from http://thechart.blogs.cnn. com/2011/10/19/more-than-1-in-10-in-u-s-take-antidepressants/

Braun-Harvey, D. (2009). Sexual health in drug and alcohol treatment: Group facilitator's manual. New York, NY: Springer Publications.

Carmody, J. & Baer, R. A. (2008). Relationships between Mindfulness practice and levels of Mindfulness, medical and psychological symptoms and well-being in a Mindfulness-based stress reduction program. Journal of Behavioral Medicine 31, 22-33.

Carmody, J., Baer, R. A., Lykins, E. L. B., Olendzki, N. (2009). An empirical study of the mechanisms of Mindfulness in a Mindfulness-based stress reduction program. Journal of Clinical Psychology 65, 613-626.

Clandinin, D. J., & Connelly, F. M. (2000). Narrative inquiry: Experience and story in qualitative research. San Francisco: Jossey-Bass.

Constantine, L., & Martinson, F. (Eds.). (1981). Children and sex: New findings, new perspectives. (First ed.). Boston. MA: Little, Brown and Company.

Courtwright, D. T. (2001). Dark paradise; A history of opiate addiction in America. Cambridge, MA: Harvard University Press

Creswell, J. W. (2014). Research design: Qualitative, quantitative, and mixed methods approaches, fourth edition. U. S.: Sage Publications, Inc.

Cushman, A. (2014). Moving into meditation; A 12-week Mindfulness program for yoga practitioners. Boston, MA: Shambala Publications.

Draganski, B., Gaser, C. Busch, V., Schuierer, G., Bogdahn, U., May, A. (2004). Changes in gray matter induced by training. Nature 427, 311-312

Encyclopedia.com. (n.d.). Retrieved on October 26, 2012 from (http://www.encyclopedia.com/doc/1G2-3407400065.html, 2012).

Earleywine, M. (2002). Understanding marijuana: A new look at the scientific evidence. Oxford: University Press.

Friedman, D. P., & Rusche, S. (1999). False messengers: How addictive drugs change the brain. Amsterdam: Harwood Academic Publishers.

Gage, F. H. (2002). Neurogenesis in the adult brain. Journal of Neuroscience 22, 612-613.

Gates, J. (2015, April 13). Resourcing. Retrieved from janicegates.com/resourcing/pdf. http://www.janicegates.com

Germer, G. K. (2009). The mindful path to self-compassion: Freeing yourself from destructive thoughts and emotions. New York: The Guilford Press. Girion, L., Glover, S., & Smith, D. (2011, September 17). Drug deaths now outnumber traffic fatalities In U. S Los Angeles Times. Retrieved April 25, 2013, from

http://articles.latimes.com/   print   2011/sept/17/local/la-me-drugs...

Hall-Flavin, D. (2015, January 1). Depression (Major depressive disorder). Retrieved March 30, 2015, from http://www.mayoclinic.org/diseasesconditions/depression/expert-answers/antidepressants/ FAQ-20058104

Hansen, E. C., (2006). Successful Qualitative Health Research: A Practical Introduction. Crows Nest, N.S.W.: Allen & Unwin.

Hanson, R. & Mendius, R. (2009). Buddha's brain the practical neuroscience of happiness, love, & wisdom. Oakland, CA: New Harbinger Publications.

Harper, C. (1998, February 1). The Neuropathology of Alcohol-specific Damage, or Does Alcohol Damage The Brain? Journal of neuropathology & experimental neurology. Retrieved March 30, 2015, from http://journals.lww.com/jneuropath/Abstract/1998/02000/The _Neuropathology_of_Alcohol_specific_Brain.1.aspx

Harper, D., & Thompson, A. (Eds.). (2012). Choosing a Qualitative Research Method: Qualitative Research Methods in Mental Health and Psychotherapy A Guide for Students and Practitioners. Hoboken, NJ: John Wiley & Sons, Ltd

Hartranet, C. (2003). The Yoga Sutra of Patanjali. Boston, MA: Shambala Publications.

Hay, L. (2004). You can heal your life. United States of America: Hay House Inc.

Holzel, B. K., Carmody, J., Vangel, M., Congleton, C., Yerramsetti, S. M. (2011). Mindfulness practice leads to increases in regional brain gray matter density. Psychiatry Research: Neuroimaging 191, 36-43.

Holzel, B. K., Ott, U., Gard, T., Hempel, H., Weygandt, M., Morgen, K., Vaitl, D. (2008). Investigation of Mindfulness meditation practitioners with voxel-based morphometry. Social Cognitive and Affective Neuroscience 3, 55-61.

IMS Institute For Healthcare and Formatics. (2012). Retrieved from http://www.imshealth.com/portal/site/ims

Joranson, D. E. (1990). Retrieved from Elsevier Science Inc.: Federal and State Regulation of Opioids, by David Joranson. Journal of Pain Management Volume 5(1): S12-S23. Copyright 1990 by the U.S. Cancer Pain Relief Committee.

Kabat-Zinn, J. (2003). Mindfulness-Based Interventions in context: Past, present, and future. Clinical psychology-science and practice. doi:10.1093/clipsy/bpg016

Kabat-Zinn, J., & University of Massachusetts Medical Center/Worcester. (1990). Full catastrophe living: Using the wisdom of your body and mind to face stress, pain, and illness. New York, NY: Delacorte Press.

Kabat-Zinn, J. (1996). Mindfulness meditation: What it is, what it isn't and its role in health care and medicine. Comparative and Psychological study on Meditation. (12)2. Eburon: Netherlands.

Kettelhack, G. (1993). How to make love while conscious: Sex & sobriety. San Francisco: HarperSanFrancisco.

Kirsch, I. (2010). The Emperor's new drugs: Exploding the antidepressant myth. New York, NY: Basic Books.

Kornfield, J. (2008). The wise heart: A guide to the universal teachings of Buddhist psychology. New York, NY: Random House.

Kuhn, C., Swartzwelder, S., & Wilson, W. (2008). Buzzed: The straight facts about the most used and abused drugs from alcohol to ecstasy. New York: W. W. Norton & Company, Inc.

Levine, N. 2007. Against the stream; A Buddhist manual for spiritual revolutionaries. New York, NY: Harper Collins.

Lord, L. M. (2011, April 26). Yoga asanas and the yamas. Retrieved from http://www.spiritvoyage.com/blog/index.php/yoga-asana-and-the-yamas/

lotus position. (n.d.). Collins English Dictionary - Complete & Unabridged 10th Edition. Retrieved August 07, 2015, from Dictionary.com website

Luders, E. (2009, May 13). Meditation May Increase Gray Matter. ScienceDaily. University of California - Los Angeles. Retrieved August 8, 2015 from

www.sciencedaily.com/releases/2009/05/090512134655. html

MRI. (n.d.)

http://surgery.about.com/od/glossaryofsurgicalterms/g/DefinitionMRI.htm?utm_term=definition%20of%20mri&utm_content=p1-main-1

Morgan, H. W. (1982). Drugs in America: A social history, 1800-1980. Syracuse: University Press.

mind-altering drug. (n.d.). The Free Dictionary. (n.d.). In TheFreeDictionary.com. Retrieved from

http://www.thefreedictionary.com/mind-altering+drug

National Institute on Alcohol Abuse and Alcoholism. (2010). Beyond hangovers. Retrieved from

http://pubs.niaaa.nih.gov/publications/Hangovers/beyondHangovers.pdf

National Institute on Drug Abuse. (2014). Retrieved from http://www.drugabuse.gov/drugs-abuse/methamphetamine

National Institute on Drug Abuse. (2015). Retrieved from http://www.drugabuse.gov/publications/drugfacts/marijuana

Office of Alcohol and Drug Education. (2008). Alcohol absorption rates. University of Notre Dame, Center for Student Health Promotion and Well-Being. Retrieved from http://oade.nd.edu/educate-yourself-alcohol/absorbtion-rate-factors/pattern. (n.d.). Dictionary.com Unabridged. Retrieved August 26, 2015, from Dictionary.com website: http://dictionary.reference.com /browse/pattern

Perelman, M. A. (2011, February 14). Anhedonia/PDOD: Overview. The Institute For Sexual Medicine. Retrieved from http://www.sexualmed.org/index.cfm/sexual-healthissues /formen/anhedoniapdod/overview/;jsessionid=C6D5B91A DB7798FC615C3AF36A71C700

Petrangello, A. (2014, June 10). The effects of alcohol on the body. Retrieved from

http://www.healthline.com/health/alcohol/effects-on-body

Phillips, R. (2014). Alcohol: a history. Chapel Hill NC: The University of North Carolina Press.

Rapkin, M. (2014, February 13). Sober Sex with Colin Farrell. Elle. Retrieved from

http://www.elle.com/culture/celebrities/a14002/colin-farrell-quotes-interview/

Rasmussen, N. (2008). On speed; The many lives of amphetamines. New York University Press New York and London

Roland, E. (2010, June). Symptoms and help from alcohol problems. School of Medicine. University of Pennsylvania. Retrieved from

http://www.med.upenn.edu/psychotherapy/user_documents/Sy mptomsAlcoholism.html

Room, R. (2014). Legalizing a market for cannabis for pleasure: Colorado, Washington, Uruguay and beyond. Addiction, 109(3), 345-346.

Rosenberg, D. (2001, July 7). The daily beast. Retrieved from http://www.thedailybeast.com/newsweek/2001/07/07/drugs-profits-vs-pain- relief.html

Salu, Y. (2013). The role of the amygdala in the development of sexual arousal. Electronic journal of Human Sexuality, 16(6). Retrieved from www.ejhs.org

Seamon, M. J., Fass, J. A., Maniscalco-Feichtl, M., & Abu-Shraie, N. A. (2007). Medical marijuana and the developing role of the pharmacist. American Journal of Health-system Pharmacy, 64(5). doi:10.2146/ajhp060471

Shuster, C. (1988). Alcohol and sexuality. New York, NY: Praeger Publishers.

Siegel, D. (2013.). Brainstorm: The power and purpose of the teenage brain. New York, NY: Penguin Group.

Siegel, D. (1999). The developing mind: How relationships and the brain interact to shape who we are. New York, NY: Guilford Press.

Social Issues Research Centre. (March, 1998). Social and cultural aspects of drinking: A report to the European commission. Retrieved from

http://www.sirc.org/publik/social_drinking.pdf

Steinhardt, S. (2011, October 19). Mary Calderone. Retrieved March 24, 2015, from http://c250.columbia.edu/c250_c elebrates/remarkable _columbians/mary_calderone.html

Surguladze, S. (2003). Neural systems underlying affective disorders: Advances in Psychiatric Treatment 9(6):446–55.doi:10.1192 /apt.9.6.446.

Tannen, D, & Alatis, J. E. (2003, Mar 20.) Language Arts & Disciplines – Retrieved from http://writing.colostate. edu/guides/page.cfm?pageid=1354&guideid=63/Georgetow n University Press, Mar 20, 2003 - Language Arts & Disciplines

Teller-Holt, G. (2013, June 1). A Phenomenological Inquiry – Exploration of compulsive sexual behaviors as an embodied experience of heterosexual women. 43-44. The Chicago School of Professional Spychology theme. (n.d.). Dictionary.com Unabridged. Retrieved August 26, 2015, from Dictionary.com website:

http://dictionary.reference.com/browse /theme

U.S. National Library of Medicine. (2015, July 28). Wernicke-Korsakoff syndrome. Medicine Plus. U.S. Department of Health and Human Services. Retrieved from

http://www.nlm.nih.gov/medlineplus/ency/article/000771.htm
  Page last updated: 28 July 2015

Voklow, N., Wang, G., Fowler, J., Thanos, P., Logan, J., Gatley, S., Gifford, A., Wong, C., Pappas, N. (2002, January 1). Brain DA D2 receptors predict reinforcing effects of stimulants in humans: Replication study. Retrieved from

http://www.readcube.com/articles/10.1002/syn.10137

Wesselman, H. B. & Kuykendall, J. (2004). Spirit medicine: Healing the sacred realms. Hay House, Inc.

Wood, R., & Synovitz, L. B. (2001, January 1). Addressing the Threats of MDMA (Ecstasy): Implications for School Health Professionals, Parents, and Community Members. Journal of School Health, 38(1).Top of Form

# APPENDIX A

1) Age:

2) Gender:

3) Age of first sexual experience:

4) Brief description of who, what, where, when, why (Detailed accounts follow in narrative)

5) Age of first time substance use:

6) Brief description of who, what, where, when, why (Detailed accounts follow in narrative)

7) Age of Sobriety:

8) Age of first Sober Sex Experience:

9) Brief description of when, where and with whom (Detailed accounts follow in narrative)

10) Age when you first began meditating:

11) Age when you first began yoga:

12) Brief description of the impact Mindfulness practices had. (Detailed accounts following narrative)

Narratives:

A) Stories from your sex life while using.

B) Stories about sobriety and your sex life.

C) Stories about Mindfulness practices and your sex life.

Take your time. You and I are the only people that will see your narrative.

I will need to begin interviews no later than Monday July 27, 2015.

The stories will be confidential. I will return all copies to you after I have compiled my results. A combined, collaborative narrative will be inserted into the completed dissertation, which will be part of the results section.

Thank you for your participation. It means a lot to me and it will benefit many sober people!

Sincerely,

Anadel Baughn Barbour

# APPENDIX B

## Labovian Structure Results

SUBJECT #P1

LABOVIAN STRUCTURE

Abstract:

Journey to Enjoyable Sex in Sobriety

• *As an active alcoholic and entering the BDSM world, my greatest sexual and romantic joy came from serving my Master and taking all his administered torture and humiliation. The more wasted I was, the more dangerous my sessions became with unknown Doms/Masters. When I was high, I ran willingly into the arms of hell.

• *Once sober, I did not care for the humiliation!

Orientation:

Person in Recovery

• *57 year-old heterosexual female.

• *Had an Abusive mother, subservient father, psyche meds at an early age, and boarding school.

BEFORE SOBRIETY

• Interested in sex at age 12 and masturbated.

• Began drug use at age 14 continued to masturbate with violent fantasies.

• Lost my virginity at 15.

• Sexual activity at age 22 escalated with escalation in alcohol consumption and hard drug use.

• Divorce, F/T BDSM, F/T drug and alcohol use. Many Doms, very subservient, even for money

AFTER SOBRIETY

• Sober sex has lots of kissing and cuddling during and afterwards. DThere is love now, kindness after pain.

Complicating Action:

Sobriety

• Sex was awful. Straight sex was the worst experience I ever had.

• BDSM was painful and I never got aroused. It was also humiliating.

Evaluation:

Wants a Solution

• Sex never improved.

• Drank again!

• Got sober again.

• Had sex with Master and BDSM felt even worse. I could not tolerate it.

• I did not have sex for 4 years after that.

Result:

• Fell in love, regular sex at 16-18. "Making Love"

• SEX=LOVE.

• "One-night-stands" to prove sexual prowess. Better Blow Jobs attracted men.

• SEX & DRUGS=LOVE

• Married, lots of drugs and alcohol, not a lot of sex

• NO SEX=NO LOVE.

• Divorce, F/T BDSM, F/T drug and alcohol use. Many Doms, very subservient, even for money. Humiliated and delusional about sexual prowess, gave up sex altogether and drank and drugged 24/7

• DRUGS =NO SEX & NO LOVE

• I feel joy from giving my body as a masochist to a sadist, beautiful form of sexual consent!

Orgasms come quickly and feel better.

• LOVE=LOVE

• SEX = SEX

• LOVE =SEX

Coda:

Impact of Mindfulness on Sex in Sobriety

• Began doing AA 12 Step Program. I Found a Higher Power.

• Age 52, 2010, began prayer and meditation.

• Age 53, began to exercise.

• Age 54 in 2012, met Peter and had the best sex of life. I consider my time with Peter the most enjoyable sex I have ever had.

SUBJECT #P2

LABOVIAN STRUCTURE

Abstract:

Journey to Enjoyable Sober Sex

• I thought I was a better lover when I was intoxicated. I think there was some truth in me feeling "less inhibited" when I was drinking, especially when initiating sex.

• I remember being so scared of so many things when I first got sober. What was scary is that I wasn't sure how to "be" as a lover.

Orientation:

Person In Recovery

• 56 year-old heterosexual female.

BEFORE SOBRIETYF

• Masturbation at around age 5 or 6

• First drink at age 7, sipping Dad's Scotch

• Mother died when she was 9, very slow, ugly cancer death

• Father sexually molested her after mother's death

• First chosen sex was intercourse in high school

- Married at age 25, still married to same man.
- Has two children 5 yrs into marriage
- Drinking daily. Xanax daily. Phenfen and diet pills off and on.
- Heart attack age 41.
- Love emotional affair with a woman age 45
- Stopped having regular sex with my husband.
- Drinking was almost 24 hours a day, no sex
- I was drinking tea infused vodka over ice from a large tumbler. All of the sudden I could not move or talk, couldn't call out to my son, and I thought I was going to die.

Complicating Action:

Sobriety

I had been practicing mindful meditation for some time before I got sober.

- One of my fears was learning how to be intimate, sexual being. Most of my adult life involved drinking.

Evaluation:

Wants a Solution

- It was interesting for me to notice in my early days of sobriety, that I was afraid of not knowing how to "be" as a sober lover.

Result:

- First sex was intercourse with boyfriend.
- SEX=LOVE.
- I associated the thoughts of being "fun," "uninhibited" and a "better lover" with alcohol.
- So I feared that I would not or could not be these things as a sober lover
- SEX & DRUGS=LOVE
- Marriage strained, no sex, no orgasms, straying mind

117

• DRUGS =NO SEX & NO LOVE

• Drinking was killing me: All of the sudden I could not move or talk, couldn't call out to my son, and I thought I was going to die.

AFTER SOBRIETY

• Having sober sex was frightening and intimidating at times, because I didn't know how it would be, how I would be.

• The discovery that "I am enough" in each and every moment is truly a gift.

• LOVE=LOVE

• SEX = SEX

• LOVE =SEX

Coda:

Impact of Mindfulness on Sex in Sobriety

• There was a confidence that came with letting the moments unfold during sober sex, without thinking that I had to "be" anything – fun, provocative

SUBJECT #P3

LABOVIAN STRUCTURE

Abstract:

Journey to Enjoyable Sex in Sobriety

• Sobriety did not take away my sexual urges. It only made them stronger. While I was using, I had a lot of sex with a lot of strangers. Once sober, I got into a relationship, but sex was awful because we have different levels of sex drive so I go outside of the relationship. It is sexually satisfying but I want more intimacy with Mark. I don't know how to do that.

Orientation:

Person in Recovery

• 61 year-old homosexual male.

• Divorced parents, step father sexually molested older sister

• Catholic upbringing, knew he was gay, hated living with his mother and stepfather.

BEFORE SOBRIETYF

• Masturbated from age 5 or 6.

• Knew I was gay, but grew up Catholic so I thought it was bad.

• Smoked pot at 13 and had sex with a boy.

• Had sex with a girl throughout High school

• Loved her, never enjoyed the sex. I snuck around to have sex with men.

• Moved to West Coast. *Out of closet and drinking and drugging and having a lot of sex.

AFTER SOBRIETY

• Mark and I were rarely having sex at all. I love him but I could not get aroused with him. I got angry and went outside the relationship.

• Meditation is keeping me in acceptance, which is helping our relationship

Complicating Action:

Sobriety

• Sober sex is dull. I lack intimacy with Mark and outside relationships only satisfy my sexual urges, not my relationship concerns.

Evaluation:

Wants a Solution

• Mark and I have gone to counseling. We have gone to doctors.

• Meditation has helped me suppress my anger and helped ease the pain of Migraines, maybe it can help with sex.

Result:

• Homosexual encounter in Jr. High while high, I Loved It.

- SEX & DRUGS=LOVE
- Had sex with a girl throughout High school
- Got loaded and had sex with men in secret
- SEX & DRUGS =ACCEPTANCE

Sobriety brought on more intense sex drive.

Partner has low sex drive and is dull in bed. *Sex outside relationship is exciting but unfulfilling.

- SEX=SEX
- Mark and I stopped having sex.
- NO SEX=NO LOVE

I am actually feeling closer to Mark than I have in a long time. That is helping me want to have sex with him.

- LOVE=LOVE
- SEX=SEX
- LOVE=SEX

Coda:

Impact of Mindfulness on Sex in Sobriety

- Mindful meditation begins to change monogamous sex. Joy and Rapture mantras have elevated the excitement a bit for me and my thoughts of love and kindness to Mark have helped me accept his vanilla sex a little more.

SUBJECT #P4

LABOVIAN STRUCTURE

Abstract:

Journey to Enjoyable Sex in Sobriety

- Lots of sex and drinking started at the age of 15 with lots of sex during high school.

• Began F/T drugs and alcohol right after high school in work place and home life. 20 years of drinking and using, job, relationships and sex s topped altogether.

• Finally got sober. Sex was scary and uncomfortable.

Orientation:

Person in Recovery

• 53 year-old heterosexual female.

• Alcoholic father, no guidance growing up.

• Drugs and sex felt good for a long time.

BEFORE SOBRIETY

• Began masturbating and dry humping at age 6. Lost my virginity at age 15. Started drinking at age 15. Loved both immensely.

• Sexual activity and drug and alcohol use escalated, in full-blown alcoholism by age 19. Moved in with men often.

• Age 35, job-hopping, car crashes, failed relationships. Sought love in Europe and found it. He and I went back and forth with tons of drinking and jails and no orgasms.

AFTER SOBRIETYD

• Sobriety brought insecurity and old behaviors. I slept around for affection and to be liked.

• After working on healing my body with yoga and my mind, and spirit through meditation, I began to like myself.

Complicating Action:

Sobriety

I was so embarrassed every time I had sex, but I had sex every time I met a man because I wanted the attention and love. I did not know how to have a relationship.

Evaluation:

Wants a Solution

• Sex did not bring intimacy.

• Sex was embarrassing and scary.

• Created messy relationships in sobriety because I relied on sex to feel love and it backfired every time!

Result:

• They made me feel wanted and loved.

• SEX=LOVE.

• I had whatever kind of sex they wanted so they would keep me around. F SEX & DRUGS=LOVE. No orgasms. No sex. Just drinking. F DRUGS=NO SEX/ NO LOVE.

• I literally hated having sex because I could not feel love around it anymore.

• SEX-SEX

• Once I connected with someone on a non-sexual but intimate level, I chose to have sober sex. It was sensual, and gentle and I was completely aware the entire time. Cuddling and kissing and can have orgasms.

• LOVE=LOVE

• LOVE=SEX

• SEX=SEX

Coda:

Impact of Mindfulness on Sex in Recovery

• Got sober at age 40.

• Began yoga at age 42 for body and breath awareness.

• At 43, began meditating, stopped sleeping with every guy that asked me out.

• Now have sober sex by choice, with awareness, and enjoyment

# APPENDIX C

## Collaborative Narrative

For those in recovery, everything old becomes new (#P2). Waking in the morning is a new experience. Free from hangovers, catching up on sleep, the experience of living takes on a new meaning. Relationships need to be reestablished (#P3). Mental and physical health issues become the focus of attention now, including sex (100% of participants). How in the world does a person do sex without being high?

The similarities were many: All four participants were sexually curious before they turned six years old with all four reporting masturbation as their first sexual experience. All four loved the feeling of that first drink or drug, so much so that they continued to chase that feeling for many years, with #P1 stating, "It's just what the doctor ordered!" and #P4 describing the feeling in this way:

> I felt that click. If you're an alcoholic, you know what I'm talking about. I ran into the bathroom and locked the door behind me. I turned on the light, stared at myself in the mirror and waited for the transformation. I was hoping my outsides would match how I was feeling inside: beautiful, loved and not a care in the world.

It is notable that 100% of the participants continued to drink for over 20 years and all four were poly-substance abusers at one time or another.

A common pattern between two of the participants was falling in love with their first sex partners. As described by (P1), "Lost my virginity at age 15, fell in love at age 16. We were "making love, for indeed love went with every caress act of intercourse." P4 stated, "I was afraid he wouldn't love me if I didn't do what he wanted." A common pattern for all four was the belief that sex and love were interchangeable. They all used drinking and drugs as the catalyst to happiness (#P1), acceptance (#P2), intimacy (#P1, #P2, #P3, #P4), friendships, talent and success (Alcoholics anonymous, 1952, p. 3). Drinking and drugs made music better, food tastier, and parties more lively. Drinking and drugs also brought shame and guilt and infidelity and violence. #P1 reported, "My drinking and coke use made me delusional in terms of my sexual prowess and I allowed myself to get into many dangerous situation all over the world, being a slave, blood and knife play, fisting, housed in a cage" while #P4 reported, I moved in with a drug dealer. Bruises, broken noses, cops and robberies were all a part of that relationship!" #P3 had legal troubles, stating, "I got busted give a blow-job to a guy in Griffith Park. The cop probably got off watching us! I was a registered sex offender until last year." #P2 explained that drinking "lead me into a downward spiral of feeling bad about myself from passing out, feeling numb or inauthentic. Which of course lead to more drinking and distancing myself from feeling bad about myself. What a vicious cycle."

It was not surprising that the end of their drinking and drugging careers, 100% of them admitted that drugs and drinking were the only things important to them. A fitting motto for all: "Live to drink, and drink to live" (#P4). Jobs and relationships and self-worth had all disappeared. Miraculously all four participant were able to get sober. The participants have all been sober for varying lengths of time. #P1 and #P2 were sober for almost six years. #P3 had 25 years of sobriety and #P4 had 13 years.

The road to recovery had similarities. #P2 had heart problems and some brain damage, describing it as "immediate memory loss" that continues today. #P4 described having dexterity problems. All described finding sex without alteration to be frightening. The journey to feeling comfortable with sex was different for each subject but the goal was the same: find a solution to enjoyable sex in sobriety. #P2 had been practice Mindfulness for many years so applying breath and body awareness was second nature, stating, "Being able to connect with my breath, both in my meditation practice and during sex was very useful for me. Meditation practice encourages me to notice the nuances of a moment." #P3 had been meditating but had not applied the techniques of Mindfulness to his sex life. Reporting that it had helped calm his anger in the past, he explained, "I am actually feeling closer to [my partner] than I have in a long time. That is helping me want to have sex with him." Mindfulness practices have helped #P1 to "have the most enjoyable sex I have ever had" and for #P4, the change in sexual behaviors was the key to better sober sex. No longer "sleeping around," she explained. "Now I have sober sex by choice, with awareness, and enjoyment."

The results of this collaborative narrative are congruent with the results from the questionnaires, interviews and the Labovian Structure results. Mindful meditation and yoga are viable and useful tools for people in recovery to begin to enjoy having sex in sobriety. The changes to the thinking mind help elevate low self-esteem and diminish shame and guilt. The physical and emotional changes to the pleasure seeking part of the brain from mediation help balance the emotional nature of sex and intimacy with a partner. The stories told showed that all participants reported positive changes to their sex lives and there general well-being due to Mindful meditation and yoga.

# APPENDIX D

## Resourcing

Resources and Yoga Breathing Exercises. (Gates, 2015, p. 1-6):

Resources create an oasis of safety and a sense of stability so that whatever arises we are able to navigate the difficult experiences with less overwhelm and more ease.

- Orienting – orienting yourself to where you are in space, location geographically and bodily, knowing where you are who you are with and where the exits are, etc., so you feel more comfortable and at ease
- Grounding– feeling where your body comes into contact with the earth, your feet, your seat, the earth beneath you, placing hands on belly center, breathing into belly
- Calling on your teachers, mentors and guides — inviting them into the space with you as you practice or teach, feeling their presence. Drawing on those streams of energy, the lineages, the teachings and the teachers as a source of support.
- Internal resource – sensations, a place in body that feels neutral or comforting, sounds, animals, a special place you go to in your imagination (ocean, mountain, your favorite chair, etc.), feelings of empowerment, inspiration, compassion
- External resource –Relying on a friend as an external resource, reaching out to them in a moment of need.

In these breathing practices we use the breath in specific ways for different effects -- particularly for supporting sympathetic / parasympathetic balance and self-- regulation.

Begin

Begin by noticing what is happening here and now. Start where you are and begin moving slowly and progressively toward balance. Never force the breath in any way, increase the length of your breath gradually and if anything does not feel appropriate for you, don't do it.

Observation

Begin by sitting or reclining and notice -- what is happening at the level of the physical body? Notice areas of openness and ease first, then areas of tension or holding.

Then feel into the quality of the breath -- the rhythm, texture and feeling of the breath as it flows in and out of the body. Notice how it changes when you bring your attention to it. What is the quality of energy that is present right now? Do you feel energized, calm, jumpy maybe?

Next bring your attention to the thinking mind what is present? What is the level of activity? Finally, touch into the emotional tone, the level of the heart. Notice what is present there. Notice the feeling quality of any emotions that are present, peel back the layer of narrative / story / analysis and notice the direct experience as sensations and feeling tones. Then bring your attention back to the whole body and feel the interconnected, interpenetrating layers of body, breath, energy, mind, and heart recognize what may be most beneficial in terms of bringing balance. Sometimes calming down is helpful and sometimes we need more energizing practices, at other times we need to simply balance and stabilize or focus and collect our energy when we feel scattered or fragmented. First notice what is happening, start where you are and begin moving slowly and progressively toward balance. Never force the breath and increase the length of your breath gradually. Keep in mind that these practices are often used in combination for specific effects and ideally tailored to each individual.

Energizing Practices

Brhamana practice

To nourish, expand, increase, energize, vitalize, tonify and awaken. Emphasize inhalation, progressively increasing inhalation and pausing after inhalation. Breathing in stages with inhalation; viloma krama.

Focus on waking the body up with large, dynamic movements, sun salutations and backward bends and postures that open the chest and upper back.

Calming Practices

Langhana practice

Calming, cooling practices that deepen stability and relaxation, increase circulation and purification.

Emphasize exhalation. Progressively lengthening exhalation and hold after exhalation. Breathing in stages with exhale; anuloma krama.

Asanas - focus on forward bends and twists.

NOTE: Often, the above two approaches are overlapping and used together. For example, if we are deeply fatigued we may use a brhamana approach to increase energy, yet end with a langhana approach to decrease heat and conserve energy.

Balancing Practices

Samana practice Balancing, stabilizing

Equal length inhalation and exhalations in pranayama and in asana. Progressively lengthening inhalations and exhalations equally. Pausing after inhale and exhale for equal ratios

Focusing practices – Integration

Cultivate a relaxed, alert focus.

Nadi Shodana (alternate nostril breathing), or full body (non--digital) pranayama, simply directing awareness and imagining breath flowing through the body

Asanas – bilateral poses, opposite arm to leg, attention to extremities, fingers and toes.

Below is an overview of the models out of which the practices for energy management come. We primarily focused on the energy body (prana maya).

The Panca Maya Model (also known as maya koshas)

These layers of our human system are interrelated. 'Maya' means 'all pervading,' what manifests on one dimension will impact the others.

## Anna Maya

The physical body, "food," the part of the body nourished by food: Bones, ligaments, joints, muscles, organs, the physical structure 'unplugged' without prana. Asana is the tool to refine the relationship between the parts of the body and maintain integrity.

## Prana Maya

The vital body, the 'energy department' of our human system, the operation of the physiological systems of our bodies. Plugging in, like electricity, prana organizes, activates and animates our physical bodies. The breath forms a bridge to the energy body and the breathing patterns are a window into it.

## Manno Maya

This is the mind and emotions, where our everyday thoughts and feelings reside, our likes and our dislikes, fears and desires. Sometimes called the 'rational mind,' the intellect, our mental faculties of perception and cognition, that part of us that takes information from the outside via the senses. Also related to our capacity to learn, education and development -- traditionally was chanting, memorization. Continuing education, listening, directing and maintaining attention, open to receiving instructions -- linked to what we are interested in. Taking care of our minds in a way that they don't crystallize with age, train, strengthen and purify our memory and belief systems. Practicing awareness exercises of where and how the emotions reside in the body.

## Vijnana Maya

Our inner intuitive capacity to understand, influenced by our past, patterns from childhood, conditioning (samskaras), personality, aspects of our character. The higher mind of discrimination, wisdom and witness consciousness. Awareness is a large part of this process of replacing dysfunctional patterns with beneficial ones. Focus attention without distraction, reduce the degree to which past conditioning distorts our perception, and connect with the inner knowing, intuition, faith, confidence and trust. When we relax the body and mind this comes through clearly.

Ananda Maya
Emotional structure, the heart, sometimes called the 'bliss body,' 'ananda' means unending joy. Has to do with what you love, what you pursue, what motivates you, being connected to that from which we came, our source. The part of us which gives our lives a sense of meaning and purpose. Asana, pranayama, chanting, meditation, relationship, ritual, prayer, visualization.

Below are Energy channels. These are the subtle energy channels through which prana flows. According to Ayurveda there are 72, 000 nadis, the following are the main three.

Ida Chandra Nadi:
The lunar channel is the main channel on the left side of the body. Has a cooling quality, changing character and represents the feminine quality. Stimulating the ida nadi through pranayama (controlling the flow of air at that nostril) cools the system down.

Pingala Surya Nadi:
The main channel on the right side of the body. Has a heating quality, and steady, unchanging character. It represents consciousness, which is unchanging and eternal. Symbolically, it represents the masculine quality.

Susumna:
The central channel located in the center of the body, from the root of the spinal column up to the crown of the head.

# APPENDIX E

## Loving-Kindness Phrases

Loving Kindness Phrases. (Hanson, & Mendius, 2009 p. 559-160, 198): The following phrases are offered during meditation as you proceed with any intimate relationships. Say them to yourself, or out loud. The phrases are for your sense of security and warmth, so feel free to language them in a way that motivates you. Find a comfortable position that you can stay in for a while, staying relaxed in your body. Be sure to incorporate Rapture and Joy into your phrases integrating them with the breath to transmit dopamine (the pleasure neurotransmitter) and evoke passion!

Loving Kindness to Self (Each line to be repeated two times):
May I be safe from inner and outer harm.
May my body be strong and vital.
May I truly be at peace.
May I live with ease.

Loving Kindness to Others (Each line to be repeated two times):
May you be safe from inner and outer harm.
May your body be strong and vital.
May you truly be at peace.
May you live with ease.

Rapture and Joy for All Intended (Each repeated as much as desired)
May rapture (bliss) arise.
May joy (happiness, contentment) arise.

# APPENDIX F

Participant Consent Form
Institute for Advanced Study of Human Sexuality
Consent for Participation in Research Study

You are invited to participate in a research study conducted by Anadel Baughn Barbour, Ph. D. (c) in partial fulfillment for the degree of Doctor of Philosophy, Human Sexuality at the Institute for Advanced Study of Human Sexuality in San Francisco, California. This study is designed to describe your experiences in relation to Sex in Sobriety using Mindfulness Practices. You were selected as a possible participant in this study because you are a sober being and a sexual being. Please read this form carefully and ask any questions you may have before agreeing to take part in the study.

If you decide to participate, you will be given a Questionnaire and participate in an interview discussing your experiences as a sober person regarding sex and sexual practices with and without the tools of Mindfulness. The study will take place in a setting of your choice. The interview will be completely confidential. No names will be used for the study to insure confidentiality.

I do not anticipate any risks to you participating in this study other than those encountered in day-to-day life. Any information that is obtained in connection with this study and that can be identified with you will remain confidential and will be disclosed only with your permission.

If you have any questions about the study or the procedures you may contact the researcher, Anadel Baughn Barbour at 2054 ½ N. Commonwealth Ave. Los Angeles, CA. 90027. Telephone 323-640-3609. E-Mail: anadel@anadelbarbour.com. If you have questions regarding your rights as a research participant, please contact the President, Dr. Ted McIlvene at The Institute for Advanced Study of Human Sexuality, 1523 Franklin Street, San Francisco, CA 94109. Telephone 415-928-1133 Extension 23. Email: drted@iashs.edu.

Your participation in this study is voluntary. If you decide to participate, you may withdraw your consent and discontinue participation at any time without penalty. If you withdraw your participation before the study is completed, any information obtained from you will be returned or destroyed.

Your signature indicates that you have read and understand the information provided on this form and that you have received a copy of this form.

I agree to participate in this study with the understanding that I may withdraw at any time.

Signature Date

Printed Name

Signature of Researcher

# APPENDIX G

Institute for Advanced Study of Human Sexuality
STATEMENT ON HUMAN RESEARCH

Considering the unique qualities of sexological research, the procedures and methodologies in the study titled Sex in Sobriety: A Qualitative Exploration of the Utilization of Mindfulness Practices for Enjoyable Sober Sex do not suggest any demonstrable risks to the participants.

Dr. Patti Britton, Chair, Dissertation Committee Date 5/22/2015

Anadel Baughn Barbour, Ph. D. (c), Researcher/Student Date 5/22/2015

To be complete, I acknowledge that the STATEMENT ON HUMAN RESEARCH includes:

1. A signed copy of the statement by the Chair of the Dissertation Committee and Researcher/Student,

2. A copy of the INFORMED CONSENT form to be used for the study, and

3. A copy of the cover page (or individual copies of the cover page) signed by each Committee member of the approved FINAL PROPOSAL.

[Items 1-3 can be sent via FAX]

[A copy of the entire Final Proposal document can be sent under separate cover to the Academic Dean]

# APPENDIX H

Institution Approval Review Board

THE INSTITUTE FOR ADVANCED STUDY OF

HUMAN SEXUALITY

A private, non-sectarian graduate school

May 22, 2015

Anadel Baughn Barbour

RE: Sex in Sobriety: A Qualitative Exploration of the Utilization of Mindfulness Practices for Enjoyable Sober Sex.

Dear Anadel:

This letter will confirm that Institutional Review Board approval was granted for your dissertation project referenced above on 5/22/2015. This approval is granted for a one-year period ending 5/22/2016. This approval applies to the use of human subjects only.

Any anticipated problems involving risk to human subjects and any serious adverse effects must be reported promptly to the Academic Dean.

IRB approval is given with the understanding that no changes may be made in the procedures to be followed nor the consent form(s) to be used until such modifications have been submitted for review and approval is granted.

Sincerely,

Dr. Patti Britton

1523 FRANKLIN STREET

SAN FRANCISCO, CALIFORNIA 94109-4522

Phone: (415) 928-1133 / Fax: (415) 928-8284

www.ingramcontent.com/pod-product-compliance
Lightning Source LLC
Chambersburg PA
CBHW041628140626
46547CB00031B/1239